THE NORDIC GUIDE TO LIVING 10 YEARS LONGER

THE NORDIC GUIDE TO LIVING 10 YEARS LONGER

10 Easy Tips for a
Happier, Healthier Life

Bertil Marklund, MD, PhD

GREYSTONE BOOKS
Vancouver/Berkeley

17 18 19 20 21   5 4 3 2 1

Greystone Books Ltd.
www.greystonebooks.com

Cataloguing data available from Library and Archives Canada
ISBN 978-1-77164-291-0 (pbk.)
ISBN 978-1-77164-292-7 (epub)

Copy editing by Jennifer D. Foster
Cover design by Brian Tong
Interior design by Nayeli Jimenez
Illustrations by Brian Tong

Printed and bound in Canada on ancient-forest-friendly paper by Friesens.

We gratefully acknowledge the support of the Canada Council for the
Arts, the British Columbia Arts Council, the Province of British Columbia
through the Book Publishing Tax Credit, and the Government of Canada
for our publishing activities.

Canadä

Greystone Books is committed to reducing the consumption of old-growth
forests in the books it publishes. This book is one step toward that goal.

CONTENTS

Introduction

'VE SPENT A lot of time over the years thinking about how one should live one's life in order to have as much time on this earth as possible. Both my parents had multiple risk factors, and unfortunately I lost them far too early. That shook me up. Would their genes have a negative impact on my health and longevity? I decided to get to the bottom of what I needed to do to enjoy as long and as healthy a life as possible.

I am a Swedish physician with over 20 years' experience in clinical patient care, working at different locations on the Swedish west coast in and around Gothenburg, and I have treated countless patients throughout the years. I have also done extensive research in areas such as family medicine and public health for more than 20 years. As a doctor and researcher, I've had access to all the research I needed, and of course, I was already quite well-informed about the issues. In the medical world, we talk a lot about risk factors that lead to disease and premature death. However, I began to think along new lines and became increasingly interested in the health promotion perspective which has been gaining popularity in Scandinavia—how to boost health rather than focusing on disease and death. I decided to study health factors instead of risk factors, to shift from the negative to the positive, with a focus on new knowledge about why some people are so healthy and live so long. I was of course also looking at many of the people around me; what was it that helps Nordic people, in particular, live long and healthy lives?

The research showed me what I wanted to know—how to stay healthy and live longer. Studies showed that the genetic component only accounts for around 25 per cent of longevity, with lifestyle coming in at 75 per cent. The figures may vary somewhat between studies, but they all indicate that lifestyle is the critical factor. This was a relatively new finding, and I was pleased to learn that I was the one in control of my longevity, not my genes. I can affect my health by shaping my own lifestyle, and the benefits are fantastic—potentially adding as many as 10 healthy years, maybe more, to my life. It is up to me to decide how I want to age—and don't want to age.

Now I want to pass on what I've learned, from a Nordic perspective, about lifestyle changes for a healthy and long life to everyone interested in improving and boosting their health and putting the brake on disease and ageing. Hopefully this little book will help you. It can be summed up as a short guide to a long life.

Why yet another self-help book?

THERE IS ALREADY a plethora of self-help books on all sorts of health conditions and lifestyle choices and how to make yourself feel better. People tend to buy books about something in their lives that they want to change, and that book is often 300–400 pages long, sometimes even more. If you're really ambitious, you might read the whole book in less than a week or so. The content is good, the advice plentiful, but the problem is that as you reach the end of the book, there is a considerable risk that you'll feel completely overwhelmed. There is so much to take in that you have to take deep breaths before you begin putting the new advice into practice.

There is a long gap between words and action—and that is a problem.

The changes you are willing to make straight away, preferably the same day or the day after, have a great chance of success. If you start thinking that you have to work yourself up to it and then begin early next week or maybe next month, then there is a major chance that there will be no change. Instead, after a while you might find yourself buying a new self-help book in the hope that it will offer some easier options.

But this book is different, and I'll tell you why.

NORDIC FOCUS

THE NORDIC COUNTRIES are known for their pared-down simplicity, and in Sweden, we refer to this as *lagom*. There is no English equivalent to this inherently Swedish word, but it is best translated as "just the right amount," and in Sweden we often say, "Just the right amount is best." Lagom can be applied to almost any situation—from the amount of coffee you'd like to how much exercise you should do—but more than that, it indicates balance and a Swedish idea of moderation. *The Nordic Guide to Living 10 Years Longer* applies this ethos to health—and I want to emphasize that to live a healthy life, you do not have to go to extremes. It's the small and simple changes that amount to a happier, healthier life.

CREATES MOTIVATION

IT IS IMPORTANT to have an answer to the question of *why* you should change your lifestyle. If the answer is that it gives you a chance to live 10 years longer, and be healthier with it, then this is hopefully a strong motivator to make a lifestyle change. Most people would want a longer and healthier life, and the basis of this book is to explain how you can achieve that.

ROOTED IN EXPERT KNOWLEDGE

ALL THE FACTS and tips in this book are based on the experience and knowledge I've gained over the years, as a doctor in primary care in the Swedish health system and as a researcher in general medicine and public health. The book's facts are also founded on extensive studies of scientific literature, health research, and statements by health experts as well as observations on the classic Nordic lifestyle.

NEW KNOWLEDGE ABOUT INFLAMMATION

THE BOOK IS based on exciting research showing that the big threat to our health is the occurrence of inflammation in the body. The common thread running through the book is how this happens, the consequences it has, and how we can protect ourselves against it.

PROMOTION AND PREVENTION

THIS BOOK IS built around 2 different perspectives. It provides suggestions on health promotion activities that you can do to feel good and stay feeling good—measures that lead to a healthy life. At the same time, it also explains how these measures will help you to stave off ill-health.

Health is not a static state. We all shuttle between good health and ill-health throughout our life.

But life is complex. You can feel good despite having a disease, while a physically fit person can experience ill-health and feel bad. We are all born different, but everyone can still do something for their health.

A health promotion perspective starts by looking at what creates and contributes to good health. This approach also involves accepting that there is no single factor that leads to health—there are numerous contributing factors, and they are all interdependent; hence, the 10 chapters in this book. The key is to activate the inherent powers that we all have in order to achieve meaningful, longer, and healthier lives—and not just to achieve good health in itself, but because good health is a resource that will help you achieve other goals in life.

This book gives advice on making body and soul feel good. And this advice is for everyone. If you already feel good, you can reinforce and retain that feeling. And if you're already suffering ill-health or disease, there is advice that can boost aspects of your lifestyle and help you move from ill-health to health, or keep your health from deteriorating further.

Plenty of simple advice— take that first step

THE MOST IMPORTANT, but perhaps also the most difficult, thing is to take the first step toward changing your lifestyle. So choose something that is relatively easy to change and get started now. Then use this book for support and as a reference book to help you add more new habits to your life 1 step at a time. The transition to a healthy lifestyle shouldn't be a chore—it should feel positive and meaningful. That way you'll stick to these new habits for the future. See yourself eating well, see yourself cycling up that long hill. It's important to create positive images of what is going to happen, as this increases the chance of it becoming a reality.

Keep returning to the book, discuss it with your friends, share your top tips. This keeps the topic of health alive.

What determines the length of your life?

As I mentioned in the introduction, we now know that your lifestyle is the most significant factor for a long and healthy life. You are very much able to influence your longevity and your health through active choices.

Before we begin with advice for good health, we first need to understand how things fit together. How can we build up and strengthen our body and mental health, so that we can feel good and protect ourselves against inflammation?

Inflammation—the big threat

THE BIG THREAT to our health is the occurrence of inflammation in the body, largely due to an unhealthy lifestyle. I'll be showing how lifestyle and inflammation are connected, how they affect our health, and how we can avoid it.

Risky inflammation is problematic because you have it all the time, but you won't know that you have it, and you therefore won't know that you are being damaged by it. You might even feel fine with your unhealthy lifestyle right now, but what may not be so clear is the high price you're paying— premature ageing! The fact that inflammation has such an impact on our health is fascinating and relatively new information that may not be known by everyone.

By how many years can life actually be extended?

DIFFERENT HEALTHY LIFESTYLE changes can give different outcomes. The figures mentioned in the book are thus averages for everyone involved in a particular study. This means that if a change in lifestyle has given an average of 7 more years of life for all those in the study, the number of years for the individuals in the group may vary from 3 to 11, for example. There is thus no way of knowing exactly what the outcome will be in each individual case, but the message is still clear: making this lifestyle change increases the chance of improving health and extending life by a number of years.

And if you make several lifestyle changes, you can't simply add up all the years of extended life for each particular change. Instead, the effects merge into each other, further increasing the likelihood of delaying diseases, feeling healthy, and extending your life.

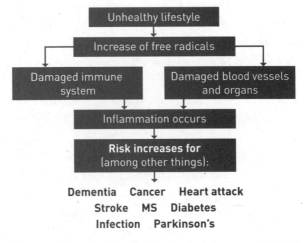

Figure 1. An unhealthy lifestyle leads to increased risk of disease.

How does inflammation occur?

INFLAMMATION CAN OCCUR in various ways, but the main cause is free radicals.

When we breathe in, oxygen enters our lungs, transfers to the blood system, and is carried off to all the cells in the body. The cells then use the oxygen to produce energy for their critical functions. This forms a by-product—free radicals. The body is able to use small amounts of free radicals, but an unhealthy lifestyle creates too many. These electrically charged substances then go on the rampage, damaging cells in the body—and causing inflammation. All cells are vulnerable to damage, in tissue, blood vessels, and various organs. Our immune system also suffers (see Figure 1).

WHAT DOES LONG-TERM INFLAMMATION CAUSE?

AS WE AGE, the damage and inflammation caused by free radicals becomes ever clearer. The immune system fails and bacteria, viruses, and cancer cells are able to multiply and spread. But damage to the immune system can also make it overambitious, so that it starts attacking the body's own normal cells. This gives rise to what are known as autoimmune diseases such as rheumatic pain, psoriasis, and inflammatory bowel disease.

Long-term inflammation also means that the body's tissue, blood vessels, and organs have sustained damage and their function will gradually deteriorate. Overall, inflammation can lead to a number of different diseases, including those named in Figure 1.

Many of our most common diseases are caused by the same thing—inflammation.

How to boost your health and combat inflammation

CHOOSING A HEALTHY lifestyle boosts your health and also stimulates the self-healing processes that in various ways combat the occurrence and harmful effects of inflammation.

1. Build up a powerful immune system—through a health-promoting and invigorating lifestyle.
2. Reduce the production of free radicals—through a preventive lifestyle.
3. Render the free radicals harmless—through a protective lifestyle.

You decide, through your lifestyle, which path you want to take toward better health.

1. BUILD UP A POWERFUL IMMUNE SYSTEM

YOUR IMMUNE SYSTEM comprises your lymph glands, spleen, and bone marrow, plus a large number of white blood cells of various kinds that patrol the body on the hunt for intruders. They defend the body against external invasion by finding and destroying harmful bacteria and viruses. They also deal with and kill off the body's cells that have been damaged by free radicals, and that risk transforming into cancer cells.

A particular type of white blood cells known as "natural killers" or "NK cells" are the immune system's special forces. As soon as they discover an intruder, they try to make cell-to-cell contact and release a toxin that forces its way into the alien cell and destroys it. That's how fantastic our body is.

We also have a large and developed immune system in the mucous membranes of the intestines, which works in partnership with the bacteria there. Foreign objects enter our body all the time as we eat and drink, and the gut's immune system can distinguish between what is harmful and what is good for our health. Good food and low levels of stress are 2 good ways to create a strong immune system in the gut.

Choosing a healthy lifestyle enables us to build up strong immune defences. The number of immune cells can be increased, along with their activity levels. This ensures that we are well-equipped to resist infections and the development of cancer.

2. REDUCE THE PRODUCTION OF FREE RADICALS

A HEALTHY LIFESTYLE means living in a way that significantly reduces the production of free radicals and thus also reduces the damage to our immune system, blood vessels, and organs. This in turn reduces inflammation and consequently also the risk of contracting a range of different diseases (see Figure 2). This book describes how a healthy lifestyle can seriously reduce the number of free radicals.

Figure 2. A healthy lifestyle protects against the most common diseases.

Smoking—by far the most significant cause of free radicals and inflammation

Smoking is one of the worst choices you can make if you want to enjoy a long and healthy life. Smoking significantly increases the occurrence of free radicals, which directly damage our blood vessels, immune system, and organs. In short, smoking leads to increased inflammation in the body.

The smoke also contains carcinogenic substances, which result in a greater incidence of lung disease, cardiovascular disease, cancer, and a whole host of other diseases. Smoking thus speeds up our ageing process, with research showing that smokers lose 8–12 years of their life on average.

Imagine being a smoker who stops smoking and instead starts living a healthier life. Since the body is able to gradually recover, you could find yourself going from -8 years of life expectancy to maybe

+8 years, potentially giving you an increased life-span of 16 years—and a healthier life at that! Perhaps knowing this can provide the motivation to take that positive leap and stop smoking.

3. RENDER THE FREE RADICALS HARMLESS

THE BODY HAS developed protection against attack from free radicals, in the form of antioxidants. Since the production of antioxidants in our body begins to tail off around the age of twenty-five, these need to be added via our food. More about that in a later chapter.

Improve your health—start today!

IF YOU HAVE, or have had, an unhealthy lifestyle, forget what has gone before. The important thing is what you do now, tomorrow, and for the rest of your life. The rejuvenating and healing process kicks in as soon as your lifestyle changes for the better, and the effects are quick to take hold. This is true whenever you choose to begin—in other words, it's never too late. It doesn't matter what you start with, the important thing is that you do something that has a positive impact on your health.

The result will be a healthier and longer life.

RESEARCH SHOWS

A MAJOR STUDY conducted in 11 European countries over the course of 12 years reported dramatic
results: a reduction in cancer mortality of 60 per
cent over the period of the study, among people
who switched to a healthier lifestyle.

The researchers also drew the conclusion that
those who lived a healthier life worked out to be 14
years younger in biological terms over the whole
length of the study.

THE GOAL OF THIS BOOK

IN THIS BOOK, I want to show the role lifestyle
has to play in strengthening the immune system
and slowing and preventing inflammation in the
body. Follow this advice and you will feel healthier and younger. It might also lead you to avoid a
number of diseases and slow the biological ageing
process.

Sweden is one of the healthiest countries in the
world, and in all of the Nordic countries there is
increasing awareness of the importance of living a
healthy lifestyle. However, the themes in this book
are wholly universal and can be applied by anyone
seeking to make a change in their life.

I hope to be able to show you how your lifestyle
can strengthen your own inherent powers. The

healthier your habits, the more years of good health you can hope to enjoy. Let us begin with one of the most critical tips—the importance of movement.

TIP 1

The importance of exercise

WE ARE DESIGNED to move about, so keeping the body active has a wide range of positive effects. In fact, some form of physical activity can cut the risk of around 30–40 diseases such as several types of cancer, cardiovascular diseases, and diabetes. And yet some people still think they have no time for exercise.

If you don't set aside time for exercise today, you'll need to set aside even more time later in life— for being ill.

Exercise not only extends life, but also gives us more energy, so we feel several years younger. People who begin to exercise or take moderate physical activity age more slowly than those who are inactive. A 60-year-old can have the body of a 40-year-old, but on the other hand, a 40-year-old can also have the body of a 60-year-old.

No matter how old you are, or what physical condition you are in, exercise will always make the body younger.

But remember that this effect only occurs as long as you continue to exercise. Exercise is a perishable item; it can't be stored in the body, but has to be repeated on a regular basis.

How can physical activity make the body younger?

PHYSICAL ACTIVITY AFFECTS the whole body, including the heart and blood vessels, the immune system, muscles, bones, and mental well-being. To build up your body, you also need to eat well. What happens is that cells are repaired, new blood vessels form for increased blood flow, heart and lung capacity rises, and stress hormone levels fall, which lead to less inflammation and a stronger immune system. Swedish doctors have for years been prescribing exercise to minimize the use of prescription drugs.

Positive effects of physical exercise include:

EXTENDED LIFE EXPECTANCY

GENERALLY SPEAKING, PHYSICAL activity leads to a longer life. Several studies have shown that regular physical activity can extend life by as much as 8 years. Research has also shown a more than 50 per cent reduction in mortality among fit and active people, compared with sedentary people.

STRESS REDUCTION

REGULAR PHYSICAL ACTIVITY reduces the symptoms of stress, which makes you feel more relaxed, healthier, and better able to deal with stress. This in turn reduces inflammation in the body and stems the ageing process.

DELAY IN DEMENTIA

RESEARCH HAS SHOWN that exercise causes a significant delay in the development of dementia. Physical activity improves long-term memory and slows ageing in the blood vessels.

RISK REDUCTION FOR DIABETES

PHYSICAL EXERCISE STRONGLY counteracts the risk factors behind diabetes-related illness and premature death.

PROTECTION AGAINST CANCER

PHYSICAL EXERCISE PROTECTS against certain forms of cancer, including breast cancer, prostate cancer, uterine cancer, and bowel cancer.

RISK REDUCTION FOR CARDIOVASCULAR DISEASE

STUDIES HAVE SHOWN that men who exercise are at half the risk of suffering a heart attack compared with those who do not exercise. Women who go walking are almost 50 per cent less likely to have a stroke than those who don't walk. People who have an active everyday life have a 30 per cent lower risk of suffering cardiovascular disease or premature death than people who have a sedentary life.

Three types of good physical activity

ANY ACTIVITY IS a good activity, as long as it is fun, your own choice, and easy to do, because then there is a better chance that you'll keep it up. The important and difficult thing is to get started and stay motivated. But by thinking about the positive effects of physical activity—reduced stress hormones, stronger immune defences, improved self-esteem, greater vitality, sharper mind, better sleep, improved productivity and happiness, and a younger body—you may begin to look forward to your walk, bike ride, or session at the gym!

To get as much as possible from your exercise, you need to remember that there are 3 basic types of physical activity: general, cardio exercise, and strength and flexibility exercises. They all affect the ageing process in different ways. Try to incorporate all 3 activities in your exercise plan.

1. GENERAL PHYSICAL ACTIVITY

THIS MEANS EVERYDAY exercise. It has a good effect and there are opportunities to do it all the time, if you think about it. Walking, gardening, window cleaning, shopping, taking the stairs instead of the elevator, leaving the car at home and going on foot or cycling—they all promote good health, and researchers increasingly stress the importance of everyday exercise. Just upping the level of general activity—without even breaking a sweat—can deliver 40 per cent of the rejuvenating effect that physical activity brings.

2. CARDIO EXERCISE

THIS MEANS ACTIVITIES that get the heart beating faster, making you short of breath, and preferably also a little sweaty. Examples of this include brisk walking and pole walking. If you choose to go jogging, a good rule of thumb is that the intensity should still allow you to talk to your running mate as you jog, but if you can sing, the pace is too low.

You can also get a good amount of exercise from activities such as dancing, badminton, tennis, football, skiing, skating, cycling, swimming, and water aerobics. It is difficult to single out a specific kind of activity that is better than the others. Choose the activity that fits you best. This type of exercise contributes a further 40 per cent to the rejuvenation that can be associated with physical activity. The Nordic countries are overall known for outdoor activities, from skiing to sailing and orienteering. The winter holiday is even officially called "Sporting Holiday" and was traditionally focused on outdoor recreation.

3. STRENGTH AND FLEXIBILITY EXERCISES

AFTER THE AGE of 30, your muscle mass slowly starts to reduce and this has to be counteracted in good time. Every percentage increase in muscle mass can add a year to your life. Building up and strengthening your muscles with weight training and then keeping them in shape can contribute 20 per cent to the overall reduction in ageing that comes from exercise. And this is an important 20 per cent, because strengthening the muscles and skeleton reduces the risk of muscle strains and joint injuries as you do the other types of physical activity.

How much should you exercise?

LITTLE AND OFTEN is the key—30 minutes of "everyday exercise" daily, according to the research. You can achieve additional health benefits by adding 20–30 minutes of running or an equivalent activity 3 times a week.

Alternatively, you can combine these activities. Muscle-building physical activity is recommended at least twice a week for the majority of the body's major muscle groups.

Children are recommended to have 60 minutes of physical activity per day.

RESEARCH SHOWS

A PERSON WHO exercises for at least 3 hours a week is biologically 10 years younger than someone who doesn't exercise.

CAN YOU HAVE TOO MUCH EXERCISE?

THE ADVICE IS not to overexercise. Research has shown that extreme training has no additional health benefits, but instead increases the risk of injury, including stress fractures. Marathon runners can suffer heart problems in the form of an irregular heart rhythm known as atrial fibrillation, as well as wear to the hips and knees. In other words, as in so many things, moderation is the key.

USE A PEDOMETER

YOU MAY FIND it stimulating to use a pedometer to see whether you're reaching the target you set for yourself. Aim for 10,000–12,000 steps over the course of a whole day, which is equivalent to walking about 4–5 miles. Less than five thousand daily steps is considered a "sedentary lifestyle."

Energy use in 30 minutes

IF YOU USE physical activity to keep control of your weight, it can be interesting to see which activities burn more or fewer calories. The figures in the table are only approximate values for energy use, as they vary depending on your weight and how you define "average" activity levels.

Table 1. Common activities and the kilocalories (kcals) burned in 30 minutes.

Gardening	150 kcals
Walking	150 kcals
Skating	250 kcals
Swimming	350 kcals
Skiing	350 kcals
Jogging/running	350 kcals

Can physical activity compensate for an otherwise sedentary life?

THE PROBLEM OF sitting still is on the rise. TV, social media, and computers are stealing more and more time, and some people are inactive for 90 per cent of their waking hours. Such a sedentary daily lifestyle has proven a serious risk factor for many of the most common diseases.

Sitting still means that our large muscle groups, particularly the buttock and leg muscles, are not used, which can lead to poor blood circulation and a reduced metabolism. This in turn leads to a rise in blood sugar levels, which causes inflammation and raises the risk of cardiovascular disease, diabetes, cancer, and premature death.

The health benefits of being active 3 times a week are thus heavily outweighed by an otherwise sedentary life.

Generally speaking, we have previously been focused on physical activity, but we are only now beginning to understand the importance of also avoiding a sedentary life.

RESEARCH SHOWS

SEVERAL MAJOR STUDIES have indicated that sitting too much (particularly with no activity at all) increases the risk of diabetes and of suffering and dying from cardiovascular disease and cancer. This has proven to be the case even with vigorous training in your spare time!

In an experiment, young, healthy men were instructed to be as physically inactive as they could for a period of 2 weeks. In just this short time, blood sugar levels were affected, fitness levels dropped, and the blood lipid count rose. This in turn increased the risk of conditions such as diabetes and cardiovascular disease.

On the ends of the chromosomes sit telomeres, which affect how we and our cells age. Studies have shown that sitting still causes the telomeres to shorten, which means a shorter life compared with people who are more active.

BREAK UP YOUR TIME SITTING STILL

TO AVOID THE issues caused by sitting still, avoid sitting for more than 30-45 minutes at a time. Stand up and move about, go and get a coffee, talk to your work colleagues, or do something else. Just stretching your legs for a few minutes is enough to counter the negative effects of sitting still.

Stand up for your health

STANDING UP AT work is the latest health trend. The knowledge that it reduces the risk of all sorts of lifestyle diseases means that more and more people are choosing to work standing up.

Many now have height-adjustable desks, so they can work standing up if they want to. Switching between standing and sitting makes the body feel better. Adopting a standing position reduces the amount of harmful blood lipids, cuts the blood sugar level, and reduces inflammation. This creates better conditions for a healthier heart and blood vessels. Shifting your weight from one leg to the other also stimulates circulation.

Standing up to work activates the body and increases the rate at which you burn energy. So if you stood for 2 hours more a day, you could reduce your weight by several pounds in 1 year.

TIP 2

Time for recovery

T HAS BEEN scientifically proven that a less stressful existence improves health. So relax your shoulders and accept that:

Life is not just about surviving, it's about thriving.

The stress response has been vital for our survival and as such is essentially a positive function. The body prepares itself for fight or flight. But in modern society, we rarely need to physically fight to survive. However, the stress response is also triggered by mental tension such as when you get angry, battle with poverty, struggle with a boring job, or have too much to do.

Stress doesn't have to be caused by real threats, either. You get the same experience of stress simply by imagining a threat or a difficult situation that doesn't actually exist and that might never happen. The body still reacts with a stress response. As such, you can sustain your stress, no matter how good life actually is, by regularly thinking about accidents that could happen to yourself or your family, potential illnesses, or similarly disturbing scenarios. News on TV and in the press constantly feeds the development of new anxieties and stresses.

We now know that stress is just as harmful as smoking. But stress is a natural part of life, and people can tolerate considerable levels of short-term stress. However, in today's society, where so many people are forever connected via e-mail, smartphone, and social media, there are enormous information flows to deal with and many decisions to make. Demands are tough in working life, the pace is fast, and stress is expanding and becoming increasingly prolonged. If you don't take time to recover, your health can be seriously damaged.

Different types of stress

SITUATIONS THAT CAUSE stress may not always be negative. It could, for instance, be something big and important, and the stress response can then give you the extra energy you need to complete the task.

Stress can also be perceived differently from person to person, and attitudes can vary when people are faced with the same situation. What 1 person sees as stressful, another might see as challenging or exciting. Different attitudes mean that some people sink into chronic stress of varying degrees, while others don't see a problem and so don't feel stressed at all.

Many find demands from other people tough to deal with, but sometimes the demands you place on yourself can bring the most stress. If you set the bar high and want everything to be perfect, that creates stress. If your self-worth is based on how you perform, it is easy to push yourself to extremes in order to feel that you are good enough. The key is to realize that your worth has nothing to do with your performance.

In certain situations, you can also become stressed by not having enough meaningful tasks or challenges in your life. Involuntary solitude, unemployment, or a lack of goals and meaning in life can create hopelessness and feelings of stress.

What happens in the body

STRESS AFFECTS THE whole body, eating up energy and consuming nutrients, draining the body's reserves. Stress hormones such as adrenaline and cortisol are released and they make blood pressure, blood sugar, and blood lipid levels rise. This increases free radicals, inflammation in the body rises, and the immune system is damaged, causing an increased risk of cardiovascular disease, diabetes, infection, and cancer. Brief periods of stress are thought not to cause damage. The harm comes with long-term or repeated stress, perhaps for weeks, months, and years.

RESEARCH SHOWS

A SWEDISH STUDY has concluded that people who suffer stress and hopelessness in middle age run a 2–3 times greater risk of later developing dementia.

A recent study showed that stressed women run a 3–5 times greater risk of developing breast cancer than unstressed women.

Some people get stressed very easily. They get angry and impatient in traffic queues, shout at motorists who overtake them, and blow up at the smallest of injustices. These people are at much greater risk of cardiovascular disease, in the form of stroke and heart attack. It is very important to invest more in recovery since stress-induced illnesses are increasing. This probably applies not only in Sweden, but quite generally in the developed world. But the stress-related condition "burnout" is almost a Swedish concept—and is very common in Sweden—making us especially aware of and apt to treating it.

Find strategies to combat your stress

EVERYDAY EXERCISE

ONE OF THE best means of recovery is to get active. When stressed, it is easy to drop physical activity to save time, but looking after your body and being as active as possible is actually particularly benefi-cial during such periods. Exercise is good because stress raises levels of stress hormones, while exer-cise breaks them down. Instead, the body releases a calming hormone, oxytocin, which gives a lovely sense of relaxation.

SLEEP REINVIGORATES

SLEEP IS NEEDED for the body and brain to recover and recharge. If you cut back on sleep because you "don't have time," you will quickly lose energy and effectiveness. You will be worse at problem solving, and you will find it more difficult to say no. In other words: you won't be able to fight the stress around you, and instead, you risk being drawn into it and becoming part of it.

BREATHE PROPERLY

BREATHING CALMLY AND methodically is per-haps humankind's most effective antistress tool.

Taking slow, deep breaths, right down to the stomach, gives the body and mind an opportunity to regroup and re-energize. Such breathing helps you to balance your inner demands concerning performance and provides space for recovery. Deep breathing increases circulation and lowers the heart rate, anxiety reduces, and the immune system is strengthened, but above all—the breathing creates a sense of well-being and an inner calm.

LEARN TO FORGIVE

YOU CAN'T CHANGE the past, and if you have made a mistake, what's done is done. Stop fretting, start forgiving yourself, and instead think: What did I learn from this? Then start afresh. It is also important to be able to accept an apology from others, forgive an injustice, and then simply let go of the problem.

Learning to forgive yourself and others reduces anxiety, tension, and thus harmful stress.

REGULAR RECOVERY

RELAXATION THROUGH MEDITATION, yoga, and mental training can effectively reduce feelings of stress. Many people find going out into the country-side or taking a walk has a calming effect. Massage has also been shown to release oxytocin, which re-duces feelings of stress. Mindfulness is about con-sciously living in the moment and not letting your thoughts drift off into stressful planning or anxiety for the future.

Give yourself days when you can "just be." Meet up with friends, laugh, and have fun. Spend time with pets. Read books, listen to music or play an instrument, sing in a choir—all this can break the stress pattern and allow you to wind down.

TAKE CONTROL

DEMANDING SITUATIONS OVER which you have little control and that you aren't sure how to handle are stressful. Taking control of your situation is an important aspect of combating your stress. There is no time to do everything, so you need to focus on what is important. The key is to find a way to sort through or reduce the number of balls you have in the air.

Write a list of what is stressing you and what needs to be done. This gives you an overall pic-ture and makes it easier to focus on what needs to be prioritized. Then cross off everything that has been done. Seeing the number of points shrink and knowing that you have achieved something gives a feeling of satisfaction. And that in turn reduces the stress.

Take control of your life.

TIME OUT

BEING REACHABLE AT all times, commenting on Facebook, and answering e-mails can take up time that isn't there. So make yourself unreachable, decide whether and when you want to have contact with the world—instead, focus and plan what you know has to be done.

LOWER THE BAR—THINK "GOOD ENOUGH"

IF PEOPLE ARE asking too much of you, it is important to take up the problem with those concerned. The person in question may not have understood how bad their demands are making you feel, and they may be open to a discussion that could lead to change.

If you are the one who has set the bar too high, you need to be self-critical and rethink. Try to see that you would feel so much better if you lowered the bar and became less stressed and irritated. Everyone around you will probably be pleased to see you happier and calmer. Doing everything perfectly comes with far too high a price.

Think "good enough"—it makes your life easier, cuts stress, and enables you to live a longer and happier life.

Sleep fortifies

SLEEPING WELL IS vital in maintaining good health. A good night's sleep greatly improves our well-being and our capacity to perform well the next day. Sleep leaves us feeling rested and makes it easier for us to concentrate and learn new things. Now scientists are beginning to realize just how important sleep is for health over the longer term, and sleep has proven to be a key lifestyle factor. Getting enough sleep can reduce the risk of a whole host of diseases.

What happens during sleep?

SLEEP IS OUR most important source of recovery, giving the body an opportunity to regain its balance after a day of exertion. When we are active during the day, we consume energy, and that puts a kind of "wear" on the body. During sleep our batteries recharge and repairs are made, but these are very much dependent on us getting enough sleep.

Our heart rate, blood pressure, breathing rate, and body temperature drop. Stress levels fall, and the number of free radicals drop, reducing inflammation in the body. At the same time, the immune system is built up and reinforced, as the body prepares for a new day of action.

RESEARCH SHOWS

SLEEP SUPPORTS A strong immune system, which reduces the risk of issues such as cardiovascular disease, diabetes, depression, and chronic fatigue syndrome. Good sleep extends our life.

What counts as enough sleep?

EIGHT HOURS OF sleep was long considered the ideal. Around 10 years ago, however, a major American study showed that:

The optimal period of sleep is 7 hours on average.

One surprising finding was that too little sleep and too much sleep were both associated with health risks. The risk of premature death was just as great for those who slept 8 hours or more as it was for those who slept 6 hours or less per night.

Sweden has internationally recognized sleep research, and a great deal has been written about sleep and its importance on the Swedish population. A Swedish study of seventy thousand women showed that both short sleepers and long sleepers ran a greater risk of premature death, particularly if they were physically inactive. Physically active long sleepers, however, had no higher mortality rate than those who slept 7 hours a night. In other words, the negative effects of too much sleep were mitigated by physical activity.

Age is a factor that has to be taken into account with regard to the need for sleep. The need for sleep reduces throughout life and is thus greatest in children and young adults. A 20-year-old might need over 8 hours of sleep, but by the age of 60 may well be fine on little more than 6 hours.

Take a nap

A STUDY OF 24,000 people showed that people who regularly slept in the afternoon ran an almost 40 per cent lower risk of suffering cardiovascular disease that led to death. It is, however, a good idea to take your nap (about 20 minutes seems to be the optimum length) in the middle of the day, so as not to interfere with your night-time sleep.

Tips for good sleep

SLEEP ROUTINE

CREATE A CLEAR sleep routine. Try to go to bed and wake up at the same time every day. This will support your biological clock and strengthen your body.

DAYLIGHT

SPEND TIME OUT in daylight, preferably in the morning. This reduces production of the sleep hormone melatonin and puts the body back on its daytime setting, ready for activity. This strengthens the biological clock and means that the evening darkness will then produce a new batch of the sleep hormone.

EXERCISE

EXERCISE RELEASES STRESS-REDUCING endorphins, which make it easier to sleep at night and improve the quality of that sleep. Exercise should, however, be avoided immediately before going to bed.

WIND DOWN

BEGIN WINDING DOWN in the evening, well before bedtime. Turn off your computer and phone. Try to put aside anything that might stress you. Write down things you need to remember for the next day. This makes it easier to stop thinking about what needs doing. Calming activities, such as reading a (not too exciting) book, are good. Practice the art of relaxing before going to bed. Make bed a work-free zone.

GOOD SLEEPING ENVIRONMENT

AIR YOUR BEDROOM and then lie on a comfortable bed in a quiet, cool, and dark room. Darkness signals to the brain that it is night and stimulates the release of the sleep hormone melatonin.

BE CAREFUL WITH CAFFEINE AND ALCOHOL

CAFFEINE AND ALCOHOL can disrupt sleep. Caffeine has a half-life in the body of 6-8 hours. This means that if you drink 2 cups of coffee in the afternoon, the caffeine equivalent to 1 cup of coffee will still be affecting the body by the evening. This can be enough to impair your ability to sleep. Alcohol might help you fall asleep, but it is terrible for helping you stay asleep. Metabolizing alcohol creates stresses in the body, which cause you to wake intermittently, resulting in poor quality sleep.

SNORING—A WARNING SIGN

AROUND 10 PER cent of those who regularly snore also suffer from sleep apnea when asleep. This entails a total constriction of the airways for a brief moment. Breathing may be interrupted for anything from a few seconds to as much as a minute.

Snoring, and particularly sleep apnea, leads to poor quality sleep, which also has a negative impact on quality of life. It will make you feel abnormally tired during the day, and you might find yourself having lapses of memory and concentration.

Sleep apnea may be associated with a number of serious illnesses. The lower oxygen level in the blood forces the heart to work harder, while stress hormones and blood pressure increase. Without treatment, the damaging effects build up and, over the long term, can lead to a number of serious medical conditions, including cardiovascular disease, stroke, high blood pressure, diabetes, and asthma. In addition, a person with sleep apnea runs a 6–7 times higher risk of being in a car accident due to tiredness.

TOP TIPS

- Try to sleep on your stomach or side.
- Try breathing aids that expand the airways (nasal strips and plastic dilators).
- If you have a cold, try a nasal spray.
- Avoid alcohol, tobacco, and sleeping pills.
- If overweight, try shedding some of that weight.

TIP 4

Sun—but not too much

Sun and vitamin D

WHEN OUT IN the sun, you are exposed to the sun's ultraviolet rays, UVA and UVB. It is the UVB rays that form the body's vitamin D when the skin cells are exposed to direct sunlight.

The sun is the best source of vitamin D. In addition to the sun, we obtain some vitamin D via our food such as oily fish (salmon, herring, mackerel, eel), eggs, and vitamin D–enriched milk. It is interesting to note that a brief moment of sunbathing in the summer provides as much vitamin D as 50 glasses of milk!

In the long, dark Swedish winter, practically no vitamin D is formed via the sun and then food becomes the key. There is a risk of vitamin D deficiency, and many diseases, including cancer and multiple sclerosis (MS), have been found to be more frequent in less sunny countries such as Sweden and Canada.

WHAT DOES VITAMIN D DO?

VITAMIN D COULD be described as a miracle molecule that is needed to keep many bodily functions working. Vitamin D is good for the nervous system and for skeletal health as it combats brittle bones (osteoporosis). It also regulates the hormone balance and improves the absorption of minerals and other vital nutrients from the gut. In addition, vitamin D activates and boosts the immune system and helps to inhibit inflammation, protecting us against a long list of diseases, including:

- various cancers
- MS
- diabetes
- rheumatoid arthritis
- depression
- psoriasis
- osteoporosis
- infections
- dementia
- blood clots in the leg.

RESEARCH SHOWS

A STUDY IN southern Sweden followed 29,000 women for 20 years and then compared their sun habits, the incidence of various diseases, and mortality. The study showed that the women who had most avoided the sun developed diabetes and blood clots, which led to twice the mortality rate over 20 years, compared with those who sunbathed. Avoiding the sun was judged to be as great a risk factor as smoking, inactivity, and being overweight when it came to cardiovascular disease and death.

In another study, researchers from centers such as Karolinska Institutet analyzed data from over 4 million patients in 13 countries. The countries were split into sunny countries—such as Spain, Australia, Singapore—and non-sunny, including Sweden and other Nordic countries, plus Canada. The conclusion was that people from sunny countries run much less of a risk of getting many cancers, including cancer of the stomach, rectum, kidneys and bladder, prostate, breast, and lungs. The reduction in risk averaged out at a little over 50 per cent. The likely reason for this remarkable result is thought to be that the sun stimulates the body's production of vitamin D.

Vitamin D from sunbathing

A SUNTAN IS tempting, and many view a tan as 1 of the main goals of the summer. But it doesn't take much UVB radiation for the body to get enough vitamin D.

In a Swedish summer, for example, getting some sun on your face and arms for a short time in the middle of the day is enough to cover your daily need of vitamin D. Nearer the equator, where the UVB radiation is stronger, an even shorter time in the sun is needed. In other words, we don't need to bake in order for our body to have enough. Instead, it just increases the risk of wrinkles and in the worst case skin cancer. More sun doesn't mean more vitamin D, as the skin shuts down production once levels have been topped up.

Vitamin D from dietary supplements

SINCE UVB RADIATION is filtered out by the atmosphere when the sun is low, in practice we only have the warmer half of the year, April and May to August and September, to produce vitamin D in decent quantities. This means that those of us who live at more northerly latitudes can't form vitamin D naturally with the sun's help in winter.

Vitamin D deficiency can shorten life, and it is 1 of the few vitamins that we risk getting too little of.

An extra supplement of vitamin D in the winter can therefore be good for your health. There is no risk of toxicity if you keep to the recommended dose. High doses over long periods can, however, have toxic effects.

The Swedish National Food Agency recommends a daily intake of 10 micrograms/400 IE (IE = international units) for children and adults. Older people over seventy-five are recommended to take a double dose, 20 micrograms/800 IE per day. The vitamin D that you make from the sun in the summer can be stored for a few weeks into the autumn, but it gradually becomes depleted. It is therefore appropriate to start taking vitamin D supplements at the autumnal equinox and stop at the spring equinox.

Sun advice

GET SOME SUN daily during the summer. The sun is in short supply at our latitude, so stock up with vitamin D. You don't have to lie on a beach in swimwear to get some sun. The sun has its beneficial vitamin D effect just as much on someone working in the garden, taking a walk, or lying in a hammock in shorts and a T-shirt.

To make sure you get your important daily dose of vitamin D, you should sunbathe for 15–20 minutes with a low SPF sunscreen. The sunscreen filters out UVB rays and so almost no vitamin D is formed. Sunbathe in the middle of the day, since the sun provides the most vitamin D when it is highest in the sky. If you work indoors all day, try to get outside at lunchtime. Combine it with a walk or have a coffee in the sun.

If you intend to stay in the sun longer than 20 minutes, sunscreen should be used, and remember: don't get burnt. Avoid showering and using soap immediately after sunbathing, as the fat-soluble vitamin D will be washed away. It takes a few hours for it to be absorbed through the skin and into the body.

Use sunglasses to protect your eyes from UV light and reduce the risk of cataracts.

A good way of boosting vitamin D in winter is, if possible, to take a holiday to a warmer climate.

Sunbathing causes more benefit than harm

SUNBATHING BOOSTS HEALTH and keeps many diseases at bay. Professor Edward Giovannucci of Harvard University reported back in 2005 that:

Thirty people die of diseases related to vitamin D deficiency for every 1 who dies of skin cancer.

But this is only true if you are careful with your sunbathing and don't burn. The risk of developing a malignant melanoma later in life is greater if you had sunburned skin as a child. If you are in a risk group for a malignant melanoma, you should also be very careful about being exposed to the sun's rays. Risk factors include being blond, ginger, or freckly, having many birthmarks, or having skin cancer in your family history. If you are in such a group, you should protect yourself against the sun and preferably with clothing, rather than sunscreen. Care should always be exercised when it comes to children's exposure to the sun.

TIP 5

Eat yourself healthy

OVER THE PAST 15 years, hundreds of thousands of new studies have been published about diet. And yet there is still a great deal of uncertainty, with the advice changing time after time. One reason for this is the difficulty in conducting and interpreting diet-related studies.

Yet, within this bulk of information, there are certain facts that researchers agree on. It is, for example, accepted that certain foods have clear links to health and to disease. "You are what you eat" is proving increasingly true. The benefits of eating properly include a longer and healthier life. Sweden has a very active national public health institute, with updated advice on healthy food. Public health is monitored regularly and measured closely, which in turn gets a lot of media attention. And there is a lot of discussion about organic produce.

Food can both protect against and create inflammation

IN THE BOOK'S introduction, I described how insidious inflammation damages the body, causing problems such as infection, cancer, cardiovascular disease, diabetes, and dementia. Recent research has shown that a particular type of food causes serious inflammation in the body by increasing the quantity of free radicals.

There are also foods that strengthen our vital immune system and that protect against and even *cure* inflammation.

These are:

1. antioxidants
2. omega-3 and omega-6 in the right proportions
3. food with a low, rather than high, glycemic index (GI)
4. fiber and probiotics.

1. ANTIOXIDANTS

FOOD CONTAINS SOMETHING called antioxidants. There are several substances that function as antioxidants, including vitamin A, vitamin B2 and B5, vitamin C, vitamin E, riboflavin, and selenium. Copper, manganese, and zinc also play an important role, not least because they are part of various compounds with an antioxidant effect. The different types of antioxidants work together as a team, so you need to consume all the types for them to have their full effect.

The body can produce its own antioxidants, but production falls away from the age of twenty-five. Antioxidants therefore need to be sourced via food and drink.

Antioxidants take care of free radicals

Free radicals attack and damage the body's cells and functions, and contribute to ageing and various kinds of disease. The antioxidants serve as a security force that tracks down the free radicals formed in the body and neutralizes them. As long as the security force is strong enough, the number of free radicals are kept to a low level in the body.

Antioxidants also protect against harmful genes

Another exciting discovery is that antioxidants can also determine whether a particular gene we are carrying will cause disease. We know that certain genes are linked to various diseases, including diabetes, Parkinson's, Alzheimer's, and various forms of cancer. Few are aware that such genes may well not cause a problem as long as they are not activated.

Free radicals are a powerful activating factor, but if the protective antioxidants prevent the free radicals from attacking, the genes can remain passive and harmless.

Which foods contain antioxidants?

Fruit and berries are a rich source of antioxidants. Go for your preferred choice and vary that choice according to the season. Choose fruit and berries of different colours according to the rainbow method to get plenty of different antioxidants (see Table 2).

Take note of the 12 types of fruit and vegetables (called the "Dirty 12") which contain so much pesticide that they should only be consumed in organic form. They are labeled "organic" in Tables 2 and Table 3. (Potatoes are also among the Dirty 12, but they don't make it onto the list of the best antioxidants below.) If there is no organic option, buy a different, nontoxic kind of fruit or vegetable instead. Sometimes there is a frozen alternative, which is a good choice. Dried fruit is also an effective way to consume plenty of antioxidants.

Table 2

Best list: fruit and berries			
apples (organic)	apricots	aronia berries (chokeberries)	bananas
blackberries	blackcurrants	blueberries	cherries
cranberries	dates	goji berries	gooseberries
grapefruit	kiwis	lemons	lingonberries
nectarines (organic)	oranges	peaches (organic)	pears
plums	pomegranates	prunes	raisins
raspberries	red grapes (organic)	sea buckthorn	strawberries (organic)

When it comes to vegetables, eat lots of them in different colours and at every meal. Choose vegetables from the list of the best, with high levels of antioxidants (see Table 3).

Table 3

Best list: vegetables			
avocado	beans	beetroot	broccoli
brussels sprouts	carrots	cauliflower	celery (organic)
cucumber (organic)	eggplant	green cabbage	iceberg lettuce
melon	onion, garlic	peas	red pepper (organic)
rhubarb	salad leaves	spinach (organic)	squash
sugar snap peas (organic)	sweet potato	tomato (organic)	white cabbage

How much fruit and vegetables should you eat?

Set yourself a target of eating fruit and vegetables at every meal. A suitable quantity per day is 18–25 ounces (e.g., 3–4 items of fruit and 2–3 portions of vegetables). To keep a proper check on the weights, it can be worth using scales occasionally.

These figures are a challenge for most people, with only 2 out of 10 Swedes consuming this amount at the moment, for example. Don't be afraid to try new berries, fruit, and vegetables, fresh or frozen—shops carry a huge range nowadays. In

Sweden there is a lot of emphasis on outdoor life, and foraging for mushrooms and berries is very common. Growing your own produce is also very popular (the huge wave of Nordic cuisine in fine dining often highlights this), and gardening is one of the most common hobbies.

Avoid heat

Most antioxidants are destroyed at temperatures between 30 degrees Celsius and 100 degrees Celsius. Cooking in a microwave, for example, eliminates practically all the antioxidants. If possible, opt for gentle stir-frying or steaming. One exception is tomatoes, which need a certain amount of cooking to release their antioxidant (lycopene). Tomato sauce, tomato purée, and tinned tomatoes are therefore particularly good.

Many herbs and spices can be rich in antioxidants.

Table 4

Best list: herbs and spices			
basil	black pepper	caraway	cardamom
cayenne pepper	chili pepper	cinnamon	cloves
curry powder	dill	ginger	mint
mustard seed	oregano	parsley	rosemary
sage	thyme	turmeric	

Of the above herbs and spices, it is worth saying that turmeric has the strongest anti-inflammatory effect. Turmeric makes up 20 per cent of curry powder. In India, for example, people eat turmeric daily and suffer 5 to 50 times fewer cancer cases (depending on the type of cancer), compared with Westerners of the same age. It is not surprising, then, that turmeric has been dubbed "Asian gold"! Note, however, that turmeric can't be absorbed through the intestinal wall unless it is mixed with pepper or ginger. Turmeric should be avoided if pregnant and breast-feeding, and an overdose can cause a number of side effects.

Superdrink with turmeric (created by Professor Stig Bengmark)

1 tbsp turmeric

1 tsp cinnamon

¼ tsp chili pepper, cayenne pepper, or black pepper

Stir the spices into 1 tbsp lemon juice, 1 tbsp apple cider vinegar, and 1 tbsp olive oil or coconut oil.

Mix in a glass with 3–7 fluid ounces black currant juice (or oat milk, water—find your favorite), drink once a day. You can also try replacing the liquid with something like oatmeal mixed with apple purée or your favorite berries for a better flavor.

NUTS ARE ALSO nutritious. They contain a range of anti-inflammatory substances and also facilitate the absorption of antioxidants. Eat a handful of nuts a day. Almonds are included in the table, but they are not actually nuts in a strictly botanical sense.

Table 5

Best list: nuts				
almonds	cashews	hazelnuts	pecans	walnuts

Look out for old walnuts, and check the best before date. They can contain large quantities of trans fats, which can damage the vascular system. Walnuts are best kept in the fridge, as they are sensitive to heat and sunlight.

Discolored or moldy nuts can contain the carcinogenic substance aflatoxin. Throw away the whole bag!

Flaxseeds are really nutritious seeds that contain antioxidants, and they can be mixed into breakfast cereals. Like other high-fiber foods they can, however, cause digestive problems in people with a sensitive gut. Eat no more than 2 tbsp of flaxseeds per day, as they can contain a small amount of toxic cyanide compounds.

Don't go overboard with pumpkin seeds, sunflower seeds, and pine nuts due to their omega-6 content.

Chocolate also contains antioxidants. The recommended kind is dark chocolate, with at least 70 per cent cocoa.

RESEARCH SHOWS

TWO RECENTLY PUBLISHED studies showed that a high chocolate intake was linked with a lower risk of both cardiovascular disease and stroke. Surprisingly, the results came from eating all forms of chocolate! For the time being, however, the recommendation of 70 per cent cocoa remains in place.

2. OMEGA-3 AND OMEGA-6 IN THE RIGHT PROPORTIONS

Omega-3

Omega-3 is a healthy polyunsaturated fatty acid that humans are unable to produce for themselves. We therefore have to source it from our food. Found primarily in fish and shellfish, omega-3 increases the quantities of the hormone-like substances eicosanoids, which in turn have a powerful anti-inflammatory effect (see Table 6).

Table 6

Best list: fish and shellfish			
anchovies	Baltic herring	herring	king crab
lobster	mackerel	mussels	prawns
rainbow trout	salmon	sardines	tuna

People who eat fish several times a week have a much lower risk of contracting many forms of cancer. Note that frozen fish loses some of its omega-3 content over time.

The Swedish National Food Agency recommends eating fish and shellfish 2–3 times a week. It warns against eating wild-caught fish from the Baltic Sea and inland lakes, since they can often contain high levels of environmental toxins (mercury, PCB, dioxin). The question of whether farmed salmon should be recommended is currently under discussion. Omega-3 can also be found in oils, seeds, nuts, and vegetables (see Table 7).

Table 7

Best list: oils, seeds, nuts, and vegetables			
avocado	chia seeds	coconut oil	cod liver oil
green cabbage	linseed oil	linseeds	olive oil
olives	rapeseed oil	spinach	walnuts

Meat and dairy products can contain good quantities of omega-3, as long as the animals have been reared outdoors and grazed on fresh grass. Eggs are also a good source of omega-3, but they should come from free-range hens.

RESEARCH SHOWS

A MAJOR SWEDISH study showed that unsaturated fats in olive and rapeseed oils cut the risk of breast cancer by almost 50 per cent. All it took to achieve this effect was to replace a tablespoon of fat (margarine) with olive or rapeseed oil.

Omega-6

Omega-6 (linoleic acid) is also a healthy polyunsaturated fatty acid, if consumed in the right quantity. We are unable to produce it ourselves, so it has to be sourced from our food. Prehistoric humans consumed more or less equal amounts of omega-3 and omega-6, which had positive health effects. As humanity has evolved, however, our eating habits have changed considerably and now our diet may contain 20 times more omega-6 than omega-3, and in this ratio omega-6 has an inflammatory effect.

Researchers believe this imbalance in our intake of fatty acids is a strong contributor to the increase in inflammation and impaired immune defences.

Note that the "organic" label means a product contains no pesticides, hormones, or antibiotics. It may, however, still be high in omega-6 and low in omega-3, so look out for the labels "grass-fed" or "rich in omega-3."

Table 8

Foods to limit, rich in omega-6
cookies, cakes, sweets, white bread
corn oil, sunflower oil, soya oil, palm oil
eggs from nonfree-range hens
hydrogenated fats (trans fats), margarine
mayonnaise, bottled dressing
meat from nongrass-fed animals
roasted onions, french fries, potato chips
sunflower seeds, sesame seeds, pumpkin seeds, pine nuts

3. FOOD WITH A LOW, RATHER THAN HIGH, GLYCEMIC INDEX (GI)

THE BODY NEEDS carbohydrates for energy. However, there are slow-release and fast-release carbohydrates. The glycemic index (GI) is a measure of how fast blood sugar levels rise after a meal (see Figure 3).

Eating food with a low glycemic index, which means slow carbohydrates (see Table 9), leads to a low/moderate rise in blood sugar levels and insulin. This in turn keeps inflammation in the body at low levels.

Food and drink that release energy quickly—fast carbohydrates (see Table 10)—have a high GI. This means blood sugar levels rise rapidly, as do insulin levels, increasing the degree of inflammation. Food with a high GI thus increases the risk of cancer, contributes to arteriosclerosis and cardiovascular diseases, and is linked with the development of diabetes and dementia.

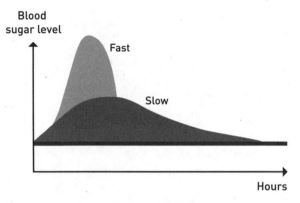

Figure 3. Fast carbohydrates (high GI) cause a spike in blood sugar levels. Slow carbohydrates (low GI) give a gentle/moderate rise in blood sugar levels.

Table 9. Food and drink with slow carbohydrates.

Best list: low GI
apples
bananas (unripe)
beans such as kidney, soya, butter (lima), haricot
berries such as blackberries, blueberries, raspberries, lingonberries, strawberries
breads such as multigrain, sourdough
brown rice
cereals such as bran, bran flakes, natural muesli

cherries
chocolate (dark, 70 per cent)
grapefruit
grapes
lemons
lentils
nuts, almonds
oatmeal
onions
oranges
peaches, plums, apricots (fresh and dried)
peanuts
pears
peas
whole-grain pasta
yogurt (natural)

Don't worry too much if you can't find specific GI values for individual foods. The figures will vary anyway depending on how the foods are prepared, and what counts is the total GI of the whole meal.

Table 10. Food and drink with fast carbohydrates.

Worst list: high GI
bananas (yellow)
beer, sweet wine
breads such as baguettes, croissants, gluten-free, burger buns, nonwhole-grain crispbreads, pitas, toast, tea cakes, flatbread, white bread

cakes, rice cakes
cereals such as Corn Flakes, oat crisp, Sugar Puffs, Rice Krispies
cookies, wafers
couscous
easy-cook rice
energy drinks, sports drinks
honey
ice cream
jam, marmalade
juice
licorice
mashed potato, baked potato, french fries
potato sticks, crisp rolls
soda
sorbet
sweets
syrup, sugar, brown sugar
waffles

4. FIBER AND PROBIOTICS

Fiber

Fiber is a carbohydrate that can't be broken down in the small intestine and thus reaches the large intestine largely unchanged. Some fiber stimulates bowel movements and makes food digestion more efficient. Other types of fiber contribute to a more even blood sugar level and lower fat content in the blood.

We have an incredible number of useful bacteria in our gut that extract vital nutrients from food and transfer them to the body to keep it fit and healthy. Eating a bacteria-friendly diet that is rich in fiber (see Table 11) can also keep our precious bacteria working in optimum partnership with our immune system.

Most Westerners eat less than half the recommended amount of fiber (e.g., 3 slices of whole-grain bread per day), which puts them at greater risk of falling ill. Increasing our fiber intake would boost our health.

RESEARCH SHOWS

A STUDY IN the U.S. monitored 75,000 women over a period of 10 years and found that eating fiber-rich whole-grain products reduced the risk of cardiovascular disease.

Higher consumption of fiber can also reduce the risk of diabetes, intestinal, bowel, and breast cancer, and can lead to a longer life.

Probiotics

The daily consumption of probiotics, which are beneficial bacteria (lactobacillus, acidophilus, and bifidobacteria), is also good for your gut flora.

Harmful bacteria can release endotoxins that cause inflammation if they enter the body. Fiber and probiotics protect against this, thus inhibiting the development of chronic diseases and extending our lives.

Probiotics can be found in acidic foods that have been fermented through exposure to bacteria and yeasts without access to air. Examples of such healthy food are sauerkraut, sour milk, and yogurt, but also in onions, tomatoes, and so on.

Table 11

Best list: high-fiber food			
Whole-grain products			
bulgur wheat	millet	natural muesli	quinoa
rye flakes	wheat germ	whole-grain bread	whole-grain cereals
whole-grain pasta	whole-grain porridge oats	whole-grain rice	
Fruit, vegetables, seeds			
artichokes	asparagus	bananas (green)	beans
brassicas	carrots	garlic	leeks
lentils	linseeds	peas	red onion

Many high-fiber products can be eaten in large quantities, but some should be eaten in moderation. The problem is that they can cause a buildup of gas, stomach swelling, and pain. People vary greatly in their reaction to different fiber products, so it is worth finding what works for you.

OTHER DIETARY ADVICE

Meat is an important source of protein—but choose wisely

Meat provides protein and many nutrients, and it is also an important source of iron. Research has, however, shown that red meat (which includes beef, pork, and lamb) increases the risk of cancer in the large intestine and bowel. The risk is even greater when it comes to processed meat products. The research has not yet pinpointed what in red meat and processed meat is behind the increased risk of these cancers. There may be several factors that interact. Those under consideration include fat, nitrites, nitrosamines, salt, viruses, and the form of iron found in meat.

Good choices are:

- chicken, turkey, and other poultry
- game
- beef from grass-fed cows.

Limit consumption of red and processed meats

The current advice in Sweden is to limit consumption of red meat to 3 normal-sized portions a week. You should also restrict your intake of processed meat. These are meat products that have been treated with nitrites, smoked, or cured in some other way. Examples include sausage, bacon, salami, smoked ham, pâté, and black pudding.

The Swedish National Food Agency recommends eating no more than five hundred grams of red meat and processed meat per week, and processed meat should account for only a small proportion of that amount.

Avoid industrially manufactured trans fats

Researchers agree on the harmful effects of hydrogenated and partially hydrogenated fats, so-called trans fats, which are industrially manufactured.

They have a negative effect on blood lipids and constitute a major risk factor for both cardiovascular disease and cancer.

Trans fats have 1 major practical advantage: they don't go rancid, and that is why they are used in many of the foods that can spend weeks and months on supermarket shelves. In other words, there are commercial motives for using these harmful trans fats.

Be careful with purchased food such as cakes, cookies, buns, wafers, mayonnaise, ice cream, pies, pasties, pizza, potato chips, and deep-fried food such as french fries.

It is important to read the list of ingredients in order to avoid trans fats. Avoid any products where the fats are labeled as "hydrogenated" or "partially hydrogenated." Hydrogenated fat may sometimes be disguised with the label "vegetable fat." A good strategy can be to choose products that specify the fats or that declare the product to be free from hydrogenated fats. Be careful with imported cakes and cookies, which can contain relatively high levels of trans fats.

RESEARCH SHOWS

DENMARK INTRODUCED RESTRICTIONS on industrially manufactured trans fats in food, and this was followed by a greater reduction in mortality from cardiovascular disease than in any other country during the same time period.

Natural trans fats

Trans fats occur naturally in produce such as nuts (look out for old walnuts), dairy products, and meat from cows and sheep. There is a debate about whether natural trans fats are as harmful as the industrially produced trans fats—the Swedish National Food Agency maintains that they are, but many researchers disagree.

Saturated fat—good or bad?

Saturated fat can be found in products such as chocolate, baked goods, ice cream, full-fat milk, butter and spreads based on butter, palm oil, coconut oil, cheese, fat, meat, and processed meat such as sausage and bacon.

Eating saturated fats has long been considered harmful. But the risk in advising low consumption of saturated fats is that we instead replace them with fast carbohydrates. This causes high insulin levels and constantly elevated blood sugar levels, which in turn cause widespread inflammation in our body and hasten the ageing process. We need instead to increase our consumption of the healthy fats and oils to make us feel full and healthy.

Recent studies show that saturated fat may not be as harmful as previously thought. Some researchers believe, for example, that butter is better for us than margarine.

When it comes to milk and dairy products, the recommendations from researchers also vary. Several studies indicate, however, that soured products such as yogurt and sour milk are preferable to regular milk due to the presence of healthy bacteria and less lactose.

TO SUM IT UP

Eat plenty of the healthy stuff and you'll be okay with the rest

This tip comes from Dr. Peter Nilsson, professor of cardiovascular research at the University of Lund in Sweden. The main thrust of his advice is that if you eat vegetables with every meal, you will be consuming antioxidants that can protect you against the free radicals formed from the rest of your diet. This means that if you let your food choices slip a little on occasion, you can still reduce the risk of harm by also eating good food at the same time.

The same is true if you eat food with a high GI. The harmful effects are reduced if at the same time you eat food with a low GI, as this brings down the overall GI value for the whole meal. If sugar is combined with other foods—particularly vegetables or nutritious fats—this delays the absorption of the sugar by the body, leveling out the blood sugar and insulin peaks and reducing the level of inflammation.

TIP 6

Choose the right drink

FOOD IS BY no means the only factor in achieving good health and a longer life. Certain drinks can also help to promote health. Of course, water is the number 1 drink for life. We can last countless days without food, but take away water or other fluids and we can only last a few days without complications occurring.

Drinking enough fluids creates a healthy environment for the whole of our body. If we take in too little fluids every day, the body will constantly be operating at a dehydrated level, which can give rise to many symptoms and diseases. Simply drinking much more fluids than we would normally on a daily basis can help us to maintain better general health. The recommended quantity of fluids per day is 6 cups.

When it comes to other drinks, the main focus is on coffee, tea, and alcohol.

Coffee

SWEDEN IS THE second-biggest coffee-drinking nation in the world (Finland is number 1)—and that's something we should hold on to. Coffee contains both caffeine and antioxidants, and several studies show that coffee has a beneficial effect on health. Caffeine is a stimulant, while antioxidants strengthen the immune system and combat inflammation.

A cup of coffee contains 100–150 milligrams of caffeine, and the effect of a single cup can last for several hours. This explains why some people can find it hard to sleep at night if they drink coffee too late in the afternoon.

There is plenty of scientific evidence that shows that in moderate amounts, 3–4 cups a day (which is a typical daily Nordic habit), coffee has a beneficial effect on health. This is perhaps a surprising finding as there is otherwise a general perception that drinking coffee is not necessarily good for you. It can therefore be recommended, as long as you like coffee and it doesn't cause stomach problems or other side effects. But be careful about coffee-based drinks that contain large quantities of sugar and saturated fat (cream, milk). Coffee drinking can also be associated with the unhealthy consumption of buns and cakes.

Since research has shown that even decaffeinated coffee has health effects, it is not entirely clear which substances in the coffee are actually good for your health. It is likely, however, that antioxidants account for the majority of the positive effect.

RESEARCH SHOWS

Reduced risk of diabetes

A large U.S. study which monitored 125,000 people over 20 years showed that increasing coffee consumption by 1 cup a day reduced the risk of diabetes, irrespective of what your coffee intake was from the start.

An even bigger study of around 450,000 people showed that those who drank 3–4 cups of coffee a day had a 25 per cent lower risk of developing diabetes than people who drank 0–2 cups of coffee a day.

Reduced risk of stroke

A study which monitored eighty thousand women over the course of 20 years found that those who drank 2–3 cups of coffee a day ran an almost 20 per cent lower risk of suffering a stroke than women who rarely drank coffee. Interestingly, decaffeinated coffee also reduced the risk of a stroke, but to a lesser degree than ordinary coffee with caffeine.

Reduced risk of Alzheimer's

A Swedish-Finnish study showed that middle-aged people who drank 3–5 cups of coffee a day had around a 60 per cent lower risk of developing Alzheimer's, compared with those who only drank 0-2 cups a day. The researchers believed the most likely explanation was that the coffee's high levels of antioxidants gave protection to the brain.

Reduced risk of Parkinson's disease
Studies have shown that caffeine can reduce the risk of developing Parkinson's disease. Those who drank 3 cups of coffee every day over a 20-year period had only half the risk of developing Parkinson's.

Reduced risk of cancer recurrence
A study in Lund, Sweden, showed that women who drank more than 2 cups of coffee a day ran less of a risk of breast cancer recurrence. Another study found that coffee drinking was linked to fewer recurrences of bowel cancer.

Tea

LIKE COFFEE, TEA contains caffeine and has a generally stimulating effect. A cup of tea contains 40-50 milligrams, which is around half the level in coffee. This is the case for black, green, and white tea. Rooibos (red bush tea) and herbal teas contain no caffeine.

Tea (black, green, and white) is also rich in antioxidants, which combat inflammation and protect the immune system. Like coffee, tea has therefore been shown to reduce the risk of stroke, diabetes, and cardiovascular disease. The amount of anti-oxidants in a cup of tea is similar to the amount in 2 apples or 7 glasses of orange juice. Herbal tea, however, does not contain large amounts of anti-oxidants. Yerba mate tea is rich in antioxidants, but with less caffeine, and is considered to have its own positive health effects.

Alcohol

THIS IS A sensitive subject, for so many reasons. Alcohol can be a help and a hindrance. Regular alcohol consumption in small quantities is thought to promote health and reduce the risk of various diseases. Too much alcohol, on the other hand, can lead to a litany of diseases and premature death. Unfortunately, consumption is not evenly spread across the population, with around 10 per cent drinking 50 per cent of the alcohol consumed. It is this 10 per cent who have the biggest problems with alcohol.

So what is the right balance? First, the positive health effects of alcohol consumption do not come until you reach the age when the risk of cardiovascular disease rises, which is in middle age. Alcohol has absolutely no positive effect on the health of younger people.

Second, the positive effect on health only applies to those who drink in moderation. It is therefore up to each of us to decide whether alcohol should be part of a health-promoting lifestyle. Drinking to get drunk wipes out any positive effects from the alcohol and instead poses a risk of alcohol abuse, with all the major medical and social problems that follow.

If a man and a woman drink the same amounts of alcohol, the woman will tend to have a higher blood alcohol level than the man. This is because when we drink alcohol, it is diluted in the water contained in our body. Women, on average, weigh less than men and therefore have less body fluid. In addition, alcohol is broken down in the liver by the same system that breaks down the female hormone estrogen, which means that the liver is slower at breaking down alcohol in women. These various factors are interdependent, which means that there are different limits for alcohol intake and high-risk consumption for men and women.

High-risk consumption is considered to be consumption that exceeds:

- for men: 14 glasses of wine per week
- for women: 9 glasses of wine per week.

High-risk wine consumption on a single occasion:

- for men: 4 glasses of wine
- for women: 3 glasses of wine.

To convert the strength of different alcoholic drinks to wine equivalents:

- 1 glass wine (5 fluid ounces) = 1 small can of strong beer (11 fluid ounces) = 1 fluid ounce strong spirit.

CAN RED WINE PROMOTE HEALTH?

RED WINE CONTAINS many polyphenols, including the superantioxidant resveratrol. It is formed in the grape's skin and seeds, which are incorporated into the fermentation process. White wine, where the skin is removed in the production process, therefore doesn't contain as many polyphenols. Resveratrol has a positive effect on genes that are known to protect healthy cells from ageing and can also impede cancer development. There are also other types of antioxidants in wine, which reduce inflammation and thus protect the immune system. Even alcohol-free wine contains antioxidants. Pinot noir appears to have the very highest levels of resveratrol, but generally speaking the darker, more rustic, and drier the wine, the more antioxidants it contains. So perhaps that explains why the French toast goes: "à votre santé"—to your health!

RESEARCH SHOWS

Reduced risk of cardiovascular disease

Several major studies indicate that a regular low to moderate intake of alcohol in middle and older age significantly reduces the risk of developing or dying from cardiovascular disease.

A report by the Swedish Agency for Health Technology Assessment and Assessment of Social Services (SBU) states that people with diabetes who regularly drink moderate amounts of alcohol run a lower risk of developing or dying from cardiovascular disease than those who do not drink alcohol.

Reduced risk of diabetes

According to a Finnish study that followed over eleven thousand pairs of twins for 20 years, moderate consumption (such as 1–2 glasses of wine a day) reduced the risk of developing diabetes by 30 per cent for men and 40 per cent for women.

Reduced risk of rheumatoid diseases

A Scandinavian study has shown a 40–50 per cent reduction in the risk of rheumatoid diseases in those who drank alcohol regularly compared with those who didn't.

Conclusion

DRINKING IN MODERATION—preferably red wine—appears to have positive health effects from middle age onward. However, reports are also coming out that question the benefits of alcohol. In other words, more research is needed to gain firmer answers.

Drinking alcohol on a daily basis can also be dubious advice, since even low to moderate intake may put some people at risk of developing a dependency. It is thus essential to remain vigilant about your relationship with alcohol.

If you are a teetotaler, you should not start drinking alcohol simply to reduce the risk of disease. Bearing in mind the downsides of alcohol, there are many less risky ways to promote health.

High-risk consumption and abuse are always harmful and contribute to a whole host of diseases, as well as premature death.

TIP 7

Keep your weight in check

ONE HEALTH ISSUE that affects many people, but is quite emotionally charged, is weight gain. A huge range of slimming books and newspaper articles about different kinds of diets have been published. But despite all the information about nutrition, diet, and the health problems associated with being overweight, the weight of the general population just keeps increasing.

Being overweight can cause many conditions that speed up the body's ageing process. Overweight and obesity are associated with increased inflammation, not least via a change in the bacterial flora of the gut, which leads to more inflammatory endotoxins spreading through the body. This in turn leads to conditions such as high blood pressure, diabetes, and cardiovascular disease. Cancer is also more prevalent in people who are overweight.

TRENDY DIETS ARE NO SOLUTION

BOTH THE SWEDISH National Board of Health and Welfare, and the Swedish Agency for Health Technology Assessment and Assessment of Social Services (SBU) have come to the conclusion that there is no magic trick to dieting—all the fad diets eventually lead back to the starting weight. Constantly gaining and losing weight stresses the body and speeds up the ageing process.

Losing weight and then maintaining your ideal weight always involves switching to a lifestyle of healthy eating and exercise that is then maintained for life.

But what is normal weight?

YOU DON'T NEED to battle to be slim, but not being overweight can add years to your life.

BMI

THE MOST COMMON way of calculating your weight is to determine your Body Mass Index (BMI), which takes account of the ratio between height and weight. (If you are very muscular, BMI is not an accurate measure.)

How to work out your BMI

Multiply your body weight in pounds by 703 and divide by your height in inches squared.

Example: A person who weighs 154 pounds and is sixty-nine inches (5 feet 9 inches) tall has a BMI of

$$\frac{154 \times 703}{69 \times 69} = 22.7$$

BMI for adults	
Underweight	Under 18.5
Normal weight	18.5–24.9
Overweight	25–29.9
Obese	30 or over

RESEARCH SHOWS

RESEARCH HAS SHOWN that abdominal fat is a different kind of fat than the type stored on the thighs, for example. The fat cells in the abdomen are active, and when stressed, fatty acids are released into the blood, causing damage to the heart, arteries, liver, and pancreas. Abdominal obesity also reduces the effectiveness of insulin and causes inflammatory substances to form. This leads to a greater risk of conditions such as cardiovascular disease, high blood pressure, stroke, diabetes, and several forms of cancer.

How to measure your stomach

An easy way to quickly check your weight is to take a measuring tape and place it around your stomach. The measuring tape should run about 1 inch below the navel. Make sure the tape is horizontal and hasn't slid up your back. Breathe out gently when taking the measurement.

Figure for men	
Under 37 inches	healthy
Between 37 and 40 inches	some health risk
Over 40 inches	clear health risk

Figure for women	
Under 31 inches	healthy
Between 31 and 35	some health risk
Over 35 inches	clear health risk

There is an increase in morbidity for every inch above the healthy value. The harmful fat is the fat that gathers around the waistline. It is more harmful to be fat around the abdomen than it is to be heavy overall.

Stomach height

A new way of measuring this harmful abdominal fat (the fat that is embedded in and around the organs in the abdomen) is to lie down and measure the height of your stomach above the floor.

How to measure the height of your stomach
Lie on your back on the floor (or some other hard surface) with your knees bent, so your back is in contact with the floor.

Place a ruler (or spirit level) horizontally over your stomach at navel height. Using another ruler, measure the height from the floor to the ruler, on your stomach. Don't hold your breath; measure at the point of gently breathing out.

Healthy figure	
For men	under 8.7 inches
For women	under 7.9 inches

Keep your weight in check— a few general tips

IT IS ALL ABOUT:

- eating and living well in a new way
- not worrying about specialist diets or slimming cures
- remembering to instead eat nutritious, tasty food, regularly and in moderation, and then the weight loss will happen naturally.

DON'T LEAVE THE TABLE STUFFED

WE HAVE LOST all control over the size of our food portions, which have doubled over the past 20 years. Muffins have become 3 times larger than they once were, and burgers have also tripled in size. These big portions have encouraged us to eat more.

A good approach to food is not to eat until absolutely full. Start by not taking such large portions. Think ⅔, so instead of 3 potatoes have 2, and so on. It is no great sacrifice, but if you add this up over a month, it could mean as many as 30-40 fewer potatoes. And that is good for your waistline! Cut up the pizza; ⅔ can be enough to give a good feeling of satisfaction, and share that giant pastry—it contains the same calories as an entire lunch!

EAT SLOWLY—DON'T HAVE SECONDS

DON'T JUST THINK about what you eat, but also how you eat. If you gulp down your food, you won't have time to feel any sense of fullness, and it will be very easy to take seconds because you'll still feel hungry. As well as causing weight gain, this will overload the digestive system, risking an upset stomach and indigestion. You will also be tired after this heavy meal.

If you instead eat slowly, chewing well, and taking time to enjoy every mouthful, you'll notice when your stomach is full and when it is time to stop eating, as the fullness signals reach the brain. These take 10–15 minutes to occur, but if you wait for this feeling of fullness, it is easier to stop yourself from taking second helpings.

MAKE GOOD FOOD CHOICES

DON'T GROCERY SHOP while hungry; otherwise, there is a risk you'll come home with fast food, instead of a meal that takes time to cook!

Gradually replace high-calorie foods with fruit and vegetables. Switch to food with a low glycemic index. This will make you feel full for longer and make you less hungry for the next meal, so you'll happily eat a small portion next time.

Drink water instead of beer and carbonated drinks.

THINK TWICE—BEFORE HAVING A PASTRY

IT CAN BE interesting to see how much you need to exercise—walk briskly/jog—to burn off a particular type of food or drink. Note, however, that the figures are approximate, as they depend on your weight and how you define a "slice" of cake, for example (see Table 12).

Table 12. How far you need to walk briskly/jog to burn off the following food or drink.

Type of food or drink	Distance
1 cup of coffee, no sugar	0 miles
5 fluid ounces low-alcohol beer	.5 miles
1 small cake	.6 miles
5 fluid ounces strong beer	.9 miles
5 fluid ounces wine	.9 miles
10 potato chips	1.2 miles
15 salted peanuts	1.2 miles
10 french fries	2.5 miles
1 Danish pastry	3.7 miles
1 burger	5 miles
1 tartlet	5 miles
1 slice of cake	5 miles
1 pizza	6.2 miles

The figures above may be something to think about before you have a slice of cake or a Danish pastry with your coffee!

Monitor your weight

WHEN TRANSFORMING YOUR lifestyle and beginning to think about a healthier weight, it is good to have a base value to start with: What do the scales say? The scales give immediate feedback about your current status and whether you need to make any corrections in one direction or the other. When you begin to change your food choices and want to check your progress after a few days, simply weigh yourself and you'll have an answer on the spot—maybe a drop of 3.5 ounces or more. Encouraged by this, you can make further lifestyle changes and then check again. This way, you'll quickly learn what you can eat and how you can live to keep yourself at the weight you want.

If at the same time you start taking exercise, you'll gain more muscle, which will actually increase your weight. In this case, your stomach measurement will provide a good indication of how your abdominal fat is reducing and being replaced by muscle instead. And all this will give you a major boost toward better health!

If you don't monitor your progress, you might find yourself eating and living in a way that allows your weight to increase by several ounces a week. If this continues week after week, and happens so gradually that you don't really notice it, suddenly you'll discover that you've gained twenty-two pounds.

In keeping your weight in check, you can eat intelligently and well all of your life, and fewer pounds may well translate into more years of life.

TOP TIPS

- Buy a good set of scales.
- Weigh yourself as a matter of routine.
- Quickly break any upward trend.
- Keep a note of your weight—set a target.

INTERMITTENT FASTING

A POPULAR TYPE of intermittent fasting is the 5:2 diet, which involves keeping your calorie intake very low for 2 days a week and eating normally on the other 5 days.

Another type of intermittent fast is the overnight fast, which means not eating between 6 pm one day and 12 noon the next.

Fasting has a positive effect on weight and diabetes, as well as on lowering blood pressure, blood sugar, and blood lipids. During fasting, the body uses existing fat as a fuel source instead of sugar. This reduces the risk of both diabetes and cardiovascular disease.

TIP 8

Oral health provides general health

Inflammation in the
gums affects vascular health

IT HAS LONG been known that there is a strong link between cardiovascular disease and high blood pressure, smoking, stress, diabetes, and obesity. There is also a correlation between poor oral health, smoking, and poor food habits. But many people were surprised when a link began to emerge between gum inflammation around the teeth and diseases of the body's vascular system. How could oral health affect the health of our arteries?

Bleeding gums—a warning signal

IT IS KNOWN that gingivitis with bleeding gums often leads to deep periodontal pockets and, in the long run, tooth loss. Serious tooth decay can also cause inflammation in and around the teeth. If these dental diseases are left unchecked, ongoing inflammation of the gums can occur, and this can cause bacteria to be constantly spread through the arteries. This inflammation thus affects not only the mouth, but also the whole body. The inflammation—which can last for weeks, months, and years—damages the blood vessels, which can cause an increased risk of heart attack and stroke.

RESEARCH SHOWS

A SWEDISH STUDY revealed that people with gum disease and tooth decay had a mortality rate that was between just over 20 and almost 50 per cent higher than people without these diseases. This was accounted for by a higher incidence of cardiovascular disease and stroke.

Being free from gum disease is estimated to add more than 6 years to your life.

How can you prevent gum disease and tooth decay?

GO TO THE dentist for regular checkups. You can then usually halt dental diseases at an early stage with fewer or more minor treatments. Swedish dentists will often also give individualized advice on oral hygiene and diet. Among other things, they teach the "2 rule": brush your teeth with 2 centimeters of fluoride toothpaste for 2 minutes at least twice a day.

Cleaning between the teeth is at least as important as brushing and should also be done on a daily basis. Depending on how close together your teeth are, there are now all sorts of different toothpicks, dental flosses, and interdental brushes that you can use. This is perhaps the most important thing you can do to prevent both gum disease and tooth decay, but it is also the easiest to forget.

Avoid snacking between meals, eating sweets, and similar treats since every time you eat, bacteria in the mouth break down sugar into acid that can burn holes in the tooth enamel. After every consumption of sugar—large or small—the acid state will last for 30 minutes. If your sugar intake amounts to just 1 sweet 6 times a day, your teeth could be exposed to acid for 3 hours in total!

This can cause tooth decay and, over time, inflamed gums.

Many medicines cause dry mouth as a side effect, and this can reduce resistance to dental diseases.

A Swedish ad encouraging the use of dental floss carried the following smart question and answer:

Question: Which teeth should you floss between? Answer: Between the teeth you want to keep!

If you bear that in mind when you're standing in front of the bathroom mirror at night, you might feel more motivated not to skip flossing between any of your teeth! Instead, you can feel good about the fact that, by keeping your gums healthy, you are protecting yourself against inflammation in your entire body.

TIP 9

Be an optimist

THE QUESTION OF whether you see the glass as half full or half empty is a simple indication of how you look at life—optimistically or pessimistically. The optimist has the positive thought "How great that there is still half left," while the pessimist focuses on the negative: "It'll soon be all gone." This attitude to life is highly significant when it comes to the impact it has on health. Not only does the optimist live longer, but the optimist also has better attention levels, a better memory, more curiosity, makes friends more easily, has more success at work, and a more enjoyable life. Feeling hope and optimism is an important factor in feeling well. We are born with a drive not just to survive, but also to live.

Why do optimists live longer?

THE OPTIMIST IS solution-driven, while the pessimist is problem-oriented. When problems or setbacks occur, optimists put their energy into resolving them and visualizing success. This sidesteps feelings of stress, frustration, and powerlessness, and thus avoids higher blood sugar levels, increased inflammation, and damage to the immune system. This in turn stems the development of cancer and cardiovascular disease. Pessimists, on the other hand, channel their energy into worrying and getting stressed, which causes increased inflammation and premature death.

RESEARCH SHOWS

A STUDY OF five thousand adults examined the participants' cardiovascular status and their level of optimism. The results showed that those with a positive view of life were twice as likely to have good heart health, compared with those who had a negative view of life. The optimists had better blood sugar and blood lipid levels.

One study followed over 120 men who had recently suffered their first heart attack. Eight years later, twenty-one of the twenty-five most pessimistic men had died, while only 6 of the twenty-five most optimistic men had died.

Seven out of 10 of those who die prematurely are pessimists.

Optimists live longer than pessimists, with studies showing a difference of up to 7 years.

WHAT CHARACTERIZES THE OPTIMIST AND THE PESSIMIST?

AN OPTIMIST ALWAYS sees a solution to every problem. A pessimist finds a problem in every solution.

An optimist says, "I can if I want."

A pessimist says, "I can't do it. I might as well give up."

An optimist says, "It's difficult, yes, but possible."

A pessimist says, "This might be possible, but it's far too difficult."

An optimist says, "What lovely weather—the sun is shining."

A pessimist says, "Today it is, but..."

The optimist creates better times.

The pessimist waits for better times.

Can you become an optimist, and if so, how?

CREATE MOTIVATION

IF YOU LEAN toward pessimism, it can be a good health strategy to try and change your attitude to life. Nobody is born a pessimist, you become one. We can learn to be unhappy, and some people practice it every day!

But we can also learn optimism and hope. However, it is not easy once you have settled into certain patterns of thought and behavior. To break this pattern, you have to be motivated to change. Thinking about the benefits—getting to live perhaps 7 years longer and being healthier, having more friends, and having more fun than before—could be a good driver of change.

START WITH SELF-AWARENESS

TAKE A STEP back. Study yourself and your reactions, be self-critical, and feel when the pessimism begins to flow. Listen to yourself when you talk about the misery in your life and the wider world, about everything that makes you angry, sad, and disappointed. Gain an awareness of how much energy you put into things that are negative or are not going to go well.

CREATE POSITIVE IMAGES

TRY, INSTEAD, TO see everything from a different angle and try to think and act in a new way. Use your energy to create positive pictures of what you have to be thankful for, what makes you happy, and what you enjoy. This is where the optimism journey begins.

THINK POSITIVELY—IN THE RIGHT WAY

THERE IS A wealth of power in being able to think positively. Say positive things and feed the brain with positive messages. But this doesn't mean you should become a dreamer with masses of unrealistic goals. An optimistic, realistic person who uses the power of thought correctly is rooted in reality and sees difficulties and problems, but rarely lets them get the optimist down. The optimist doesn't try to ignore the negative—but is not hamstrung by it and always works to change and convert the negative into something positive. The optimist hopes for the best, but is prepared for the worst.

EXPRESS GRATITUDE AND JOY

ACKNOWLEDGE WHAT IS meaningful in your life and embrace everything around you that is good. Express gratitude and joy for the big things and the small. What this generates is a general level of "everyday happiness." The optimist sees this and is filled with positive emotions.

SURROUND YOURSELF WITH POSITIVE PEOPLE

YOU ARE WHO you spend time with. Avoid pessimists who drain your energy. Instead, socialize in circles where the optimists can be found. They radiate energy—it's infectious. Then share your positive energy with your nearest and dearest. This will create *joie de vivre* and health for both you and those around you.

LAUGH AND SMILE

HUMOR AND LAUGHTER reduce stress hormones, lower blood pressure, and improve your mood. Laughing increases the level of endorphins, giving feelings of pleasure and reward. Feelings of stress disappear, inflammation in the body reduces, and the immune system becomes stronger and more effective. There really is something in the old saying, "Laughter is the best medicine." Act like a happy person, walk around with a spring in your step and a smile on your lips, and this will cheer you up.

BE PHYSICALLY ACTIVE

PHYSICAL ACTIVITY OF various kinds burns up stress hormones and releases the feel-good hormone dopamine. This creates a sense of well-being that makes it easier to think positive thoughts.

BE GENEROUS TOWARD OTHERS

AT HEART, PEOPLE are givers, and we get more pleasure from giving than from receiving. So give your energy and time freely. If you are in the habit of giving a helping hand to someone who needs it, of being there for a friend, that is an important source of positive feelings. Be just as enthusiastic about other people's successes as you are about your own.

TIP 10

We need each other

PEOPLE ARE PACK animals—we need each other. There is a deep-seated need for social relationships and human support in order to survive and stay healthy. Social intercourse may well have been one of the key strategies for the survival of the human race.

At the heart of a harmonious existence lies good family relationships, work colleagues, and a stable circle of friends. But it is not the number of friends and social encounters that is important, it is their quality. Good relationships with a few are better than many relationships of poor quality.

You can feel alone even when you are surrounded by people, either as a couple or a group. Everyone is alone sometimes, and it is normal to feel lonely. Self-imposed solitude is not associated with any health risk. The problem is with involuntary loneliness.

AVOID ENERGY THIEVES

GOOD RELATIONSHIPS CREATE positive energy that promotes health and well-being. However, the opposite is also true, with some people around you stealing your energy. After such an encounter, you can feel tired, drained, and a bit of a failure. Choose the right friends and foster a healthy social life.

WHAT DO YOU GAIN FROM TIME WITH FRIENDS?

EVERYTHING THAT PROMOTES feelings of inclusion and social belonging and that makes you feel respected and liked for who you are—and being able to give the same back—is good for you. The more we share with each other, the healthier and stronger we and our relationships are.

A good social life has a positive effect in that it boosts the feel-good hormone, reduces the stress hormones, and thereby also decreases inflammation. Our immune system is strengthened and this leads to a longer life, with more fun in it.

You may be strong on your own, but being part of a positive social circle makes you even stronger.

Those who live in positive relationships—with good, close relatives, friends, or a beloved pet—recover faster from illness and live longer.

RESEARCH SHOWS

SEVERAL STUDIES HAVE shown higher mortality rates among individuals who are lonely. For example, a person living alone has a higher risk of dying from a stroke than people living together.

In a large study of 180,000 people, the risk of a heart attack rose by almost 30 per cent in those who felt lonely or had few social contacts. The corresponding figure for stroke was an increased risk of just over 30 per cent.

A U.S. study showed that the risk of developing Alzheimer's was more than twice as great for those who felt lonely, compared with those who didn't.

THE DANGERS OF LONELINESS

IF SOCIAL RELATIONSHIPS are insufficient over a prolonged period, the vulnerability of the individual increases. The dangers of loneliness arise from not having anyone to share your feelings with or to have close contact with. Loneliness can cause more suffering than physical pain.

Sometimes those around you help to make the loneliness feel even worse. One example is the elated grandmother who talks and talks about her fantastic children, not to mention her even more incredible grandchildren. She doesn't think for a second that there may be someone listening in the group who doesn't have any family or whose childlessness was not a choice. It is thus important to be aware of the situation you are in and to think about what you say, so as not to hurt anyone. It is also important to be on the lookout for anyone, for example at work, who feels excluded from the social group. In such a case, it is good to be generous, to show engagement with and interest in the person in question, invite the person for a chat, and see a friendship develop.

Our social environment has crucial consequences for our health. If you feel lonely, excluded, and without support, your resistance to stress and disease is reduced. Psychological stress creates inflammation and has a direct harmful effect on the immune system, the cardiovascular system, and the body's other organs. This raises the risk of illness and a shorter life.

Many people are well aware that stress, obesity, and sitting still are harmful to health, but it is much less well-known that involuntary loneliness can be a major factor in ill-health. The advice in this chapter therefore delves more deeply into ways of shaking off loneliness, something that is largely an internal process.

The dangers of loneliness double the risk of falling ill and dying. Feeling excluded affects mortality just as much as—or more than—smoking, stress, obesity, or high blood pressure.

DEVELOP FRIENDSHIPS

DEVELOPING FRIENDSHIP TAKES time, and friendship has to be nurtured and maintained. You have to care, make contact, and listen. The friendship will then deepen over time and become a source of joy and trust. To establish a good relationship with other people, it is important to:

- speak from the heart, be able to talk about topics large and small, and be a good listener
- be positive, show appreciation, give feedback, and have fun together
- show consideration
- respect each other's differences, be able to compromise, and be flexible.

When it comes to that wonderful, genuine meeting between people, it is important to feel and show empathy—to always try to put yourself in the other person's shoes. If you don't know where the person is coming from, you can't properly be a good friend and show mutual respect. Nor can you give support or advice, if the need arises. Keeping this in mind as you develop your network of close friends will make those friendships deep, lasting, and enriching.

HOW DO YOU FIND NEW FRIENDS?

FRIENDSHIPS CAN BE created in many different ways and they don't have to be age-dependent.
Friends of different ages make life richer. Everyone
has opportunities to find new friends, whatever
their situation. In Sweden there is a widespread and
diverse culture of sporting clubs and hobby circles,
which are partly subsidized by the government.

Contacts can be made by:

- attending a course or joining a club that
interests you such as a cooking course, a pho-
tography course, birdwatching, a gardening
club, or a sports club—where you'll meet like-
minded people
- having the courage to travel alone and talk to
people you don't know
- going out dancing
- using social media such as Facebook, chat
rooms, online dating sites
- taking up walking, exercise, or aerobics with
someone
- inviting a neighbor round for coffee or going to
the movies with someone
- getting involved in community organizations
- singing in a choir
- having a beloved pet as a friend.

MAKING FRIENDS ISN'T EASY

THERE ARE ALL sorts of obstacles that can stop friendships from happening. The most common of these are:

- Fear: the prospect of meeting new people can be both exciting and terrifying. Fear often wins out over curiosity.
- Low self-esteem: "Why would anyone want to spend time with me? I have nothing to offer, and everyone is bound to find me boring."
- An unsafe neighborhood and fear of going out alone at night. This can stop you from getting out and meeting people.

Fear and low self-esteem lead people to make poor decisions. Despite being unhappy about the loneliness, they can't pluck up the courage to do anything about it.

THE KEYS TO CHANGE

Step 1—understanding

The first step is to understand your situation, be honest with yourself, clearly see the problem, and understand its consequences.

"I'm lonely. I don't have any really good friends or a life partner. I sit here all alone on a Friday night, while others have cosy evenings together. The big holidays are the saddest days of the year, when the loneliness is particularly painful. I'm often sad, and it feels like life is just passing me by."

It can be really tough to put together this picture of yourself and really understand your situation. But this is how you enable change, as in this moment of clarity you may realize that something has to be done.

Step 2—create motivation

And so the ideas come thick and fast about maybe trying something new. This creates motivation, and that is the wave of energy that will lead you to take action to break the cycle of loneliness.

Each individual will usually have a personal solution to the problem—something that suits the individual's particular situation. The best solution is there—inside of you.

In this phase, you have to overcome your fears— "What if I embarrass myself? What if something happens to me as I walk home in the dark? What if I get tricked by someone on social media?" Fear is a defence mechanism that can make life very limited. But now you have to let go, dare to move on. You should still be critically assessing the various alternatives, but don't exaggerate the dangers. Instead, paint a positive picture of what you want to achieve.

Step 3—set up a goal

You now have the motivation and drive to change your situation, and so you need to immediately set up your goal: What do I want my life to look like and how can I achieve that? What do I need to do first? What should I try? Now you're on the right track—a goal has been set and a decision made.

Step 4—take the initiative

And now for action—finally there is a chance of something happening. Naturally, there are friends or a good partner out there for you; you just need the energy and the focus to find the "treasure"—because having friends and leading a longer, healthier, and more fun life truly is a treasure.

DON'T GIVE UP

IF ANXIETY AND insecurity arise, take stock of your current situation. This is what my life is like today—do I want to keep living this way? The answer is no, so embrace your vision again and overcome the fear. It's time for things to start happening. Don't think, "How is it going to go?" but, "What must I do to make it go well?"

There are plenty of lovely little cards available with sayings and messages about daring to take the first step, believing in yourself, you can do it, you are worth it, and so on. These affirmations can be placed on the bathroom mirror or the fridge, for example, as a reminder of this new self-image and that you are going to succeed.

Once you've taken a first step, you've set things in motion and then it's easy to think, "Now I'm going to take the next step." It becomes a positive spiral, after that most difficult first step.

Of course, there will be days when you start to doubt yourself, and feel tired and vulnerable. Maybe that day you won't take a step forward, but it is important to keep your goal in mind and get started again as soon as possible. Don't give up at the first hurdle and, instead, maybe try being even more flexible about the way you achieve your goal. If your first attempt doesn't go well, think of a new, possibly better, solution.

If a setback can be seen as a valuable and important experience, this increases the chance of things going better next time. Setbacks are good as they offer an opportunity to grow and develop. An unwillingness to fail comes down to fear. But let your curiosity prevail, instead. Uncertainty is part of life, the part that makes it exciting. Spread your wings, dare to succeed!

Start today!

THIS BOOK MAY have come to an end, but the rest of your life has just begun! How are you going to live it?

Now you know what makes you stronger and what slows the ageing process.

You have the chance to change your lifestyle, so my final tip is: start today—or tomorrow.

Good luck!

FACTS AND REFERENCES

———————————

THE BOOK'S FACTS are all based on the knowledge and experience that I have gained from my 20 years as a doctor in primary care and then 20 years as a researcher into general medicine and public health at the University of Gothenburg.

The book's facts are also based on a large number of scientific articles, systematic summaries of research results, reference books, and national guidelines and statements by established and respected researchers and authors.

Bibliography

General references with links to multiple chapters in the book.

Antonovsky, A. *Hälsans mysterium* (*Health's Mystery*), 2nd edition. Stockholm: Natur & Kultur, 2005. (*Unraveling the Mystery of Health*. San Francisco: Jossey-Bass Inc., 1987).

Carper, J. *Mirakelhjärnan* (*The Miracle Brain*), 2nd edition. Stockholm: Forum, 2001.

Csíkszentmihályi, M. *Finna flow, den vardagliga entusiasmens psykologi* (*Find Flow: The Psychology of Everyday Enthusiasm*). Stockholm: Natur & Kultur, 1999.

Ehdin Anandala, S. *Nya självläkande människan* (*The New Self-healing Human*), 2nd edition. Stockholm: Bladh by Bladh, 2014.

Ennart, H. *Åldrandets gåta, metoderna som förlänger ditt liv* (*The Riddle of Ageing: Methods that Extend Your Life*). Stockholm: Ordfront, 2013.

Marklund, B., *Symtom, Råd, Åtgärd* (*Symptoms, Advice, Action*), 9th edition. Lund: Studentlitteratur, 2008.

Roizen, M. *RealAge: Are You as Young as You Can Be?* HarperCollins e-book, 2010.

Servan-Schreiber, D. *Anticancer, ett nytt sätt att leva* (*Anticancer: A New Way of Life*). Stockholm: Natur & Kultur, 2011.

World Health Organization. *Ottawa Charter for Health Promotion*. Copenhagen: WHO Regional Office for Europe, 1986.

Specific references with links to particular chapters in the book.

What determines the length of your life?

Khaw, K. T. et al. "Combined Impact of Health Behaviours and Mortality in Men and Women: The EPIC-Norfolk Prospective Population Study." *PLOS Medicine* 5(1): e12 (2008).

Knoops, K.T.B. et al. "Mediterranean Diet, Lifestyle Factors, and 10-Year Mortality in Elderly European Men and Women: The HALE Project." *Journal of the American Medical Association* 292, no. 12 (2004): 1433–39.

Lichtenstein, P. et al. "Environmental and Heritable Factors in the Causation of Cancer–Analyses of Cohorts of Twins from Sweden, Denmark, and Finland." *New England Journal of Medicine* 343, no. 2 (2000): 78–85.

Wilhelmsen, L. et al. "Factors Associated with Reaching 90 Years of Age: A Study of Men Born in 1913 in Gothenburg, Sweden." *Journal of Internal Medicine* 269, no. 4 (2011): 441–51.

Tip 1. The importance of exercise

Biswas, A. et al. "Sedentary Time and Its Association with Risk for Disease Incidence, Mortality, and Hospitalization in Adults: A Systematic Review and Meta-analysis." *Annals of Internal Medicine* 162, no. 2 (2015): 123–32.

Dunstan, D.W. et al. "Television Viewing Time and Mortality: The Australian Diabetes, Obesity and Lifestyle Study." *Circulation* 121, no. 3 (2010): 384–91.

Fröberg, A. and Raustorp, A. "Samband mellan stillasittande och ohälsa varierar med mätmetod" ("Correlation Between Sitting Still and Ill-Health Varies with Measurement Method"). *Läkartidningen* 113 (2016): DU33.

Henriksson, J. et al. FYSS: *Fysisk aktivitet i sjukdomsprevention och sjukdomsbehandling* (*Physical Activity in the Prevention and Treatment of Disease*). Swedish National Institute of Public Health (2003).

Jansson, E. et al. "Fysisk aktivitet: nya vägar och val i rekommendationerna för vuxna" ("Physical Activity: New Paths and Options in Recommendations for Adults"). *Läkartidningen* 112 (2015): DP7W.

Johansson, S. and Qvist, J. "Motion förlänger livet" ("Exercise Extends Life"). *Välfärdsbulletinen* 2 (1997): 12.

Norling, I. et al. *Fritid och hälsa (Recreation and Health)*, Report 11. Gothenburg: Research and Development Unit, Lövgärdet, 1995.

Senchina, D.S. "Effects of Regular Exercise on the Aging Immune System: A Review." *Clinical Journal of Sport Medicine* 19, no. 5 (2009): 439–40.

Smith, T.C. et al. "Walking Decreased Risk of Cardiovascular Disease Mortality in Older Adults with Diabetes." *Journal of Clinical Epidemiology* 60, no.3 (2007): 309–17.

Sundberg, C. J. and Jansson, E. "Fysisk aktivitet en viktig medicin" ("Physical Activity an Important Medicine"). *Läkartidningen* 112 (2015): DRT4.

Tip 2. Time for recovery

Arnetz, B. and Ekman, R. (eds.). *Stress: Gen, Individ, Samhälle (Stress: Gene, Individual, Society)*, 3rd edition. Stockholm: Liber AB, 2013.

Kivipelto, M. et al. "A 2 Year Multidomain Intervention of Diet, Exercise, Cognitive Training, and Vascular Risk Monitoring Versus Control to Prevent Cognitive Decline in At-Risk Elderly People (FINGER): A Randomised Controlled Trial." *Lancet* 385, no. 9984 (2015): 2255–63.

Melander, O. et al. "Stable Peptide of the Endogenous
    Opioid Enkephalin Precursor and Breast Cancer Risk."
    Journal of Clinical Oncology 33, no. 24 (2015): 2632–38.

Tip 3. Sleep fortifies

Åkerstedt, T. "Livsstilen påverkar sömnen—på gott och ont"
    ("Lifestyle Affects Sleep—for Good and Bad"). *Läkartid-*
    ningen 107 (2010): 2072–76.

Bellavia, A. et al. "Sleep Duration and Survival Percentiles
    Across Categories of Physical Activity." *American Jour-*
    nal of Epidemiology 179, no. 4 (2014): 484–91.

Kripke, D. et al. "Mortality Associated with Sleep Duration
    and Insomnia." *Archives of General Psychiatry* 59,
    no. 2 (2002): 131–36.

Naska, A. et al. "Siesta in Healthy Adults and Coronary
    Mortality in the General Population." *Archives of Inter-*
    nal Medicine 167, no. 3 (2007): 296–301.

Tip 4. Sun—but not too much

Giovannucci, E. Speech at the American Association for
    Cancer Research conference in Anaheim, California,
    2005.

Giovannucci, E. "Vitamin D Status and Cancer Incidence
    and Mortality." *Advances in Experimental Medicine*
    and Biology 624 (2008): 31–42.

Lindqvist, P.G. et al. "Avoidance of Sun Exposure as a Risk
    Factor for Major Causes of Death: A Competing Risk
    Analysis of the Melanoma in Southern Sweden Cohort."
    Journal of Internal Medicine 280, no. 4 (2016): 375–87.

Tuohimaa, P. et al. "Does Solar Exposure, as Indicated by the Non-Melanoma Skin Cancers, Protect from Solid Cancers: Vitamin D as a Possible Explanation." *European Journal of Cancer* 43, no. 11 (2007): 1701–12.

Tip 5. Eat yourself healthy

Bengmark, S. "Den bioekologiska medicinen har kommit för att stanna. Om flora, synbiotika, immunitet och resistens mot sjukdom" ("Bioecological Medicine Is Here to Stay. On Flora, Symbiotics, Immunity and Resistance to Disease"). *Läkartidningen* 102 (2005): 2–6.

Bengmark, S. "Vår tids kost bakom inflammation och sjukdomsutveckling" ("Modern Diet Behind Inflammation and Disease Development"). *Läkartidningen* 104 (2007): 3873–77.

Cederholm, T. and Hellénius, M. L. "Matens betydelse för åldrande och livslängd" ("The Importance of Nutrition for Aging and Longevity"). *Läkartidningen* 113 (2016): DYMA.

Cederholm, T. and Rothenberg, E. "Krypskytte mot vetenskapen äventyrar folkhälsoarbetet ("Sniping Against Science Jeopardizes Public Health Work"). *Läkartidningen* 113 (2016): 784–85.

Knoops, K.T. et al. "Mediterranean Diet, Lifestyle Factors, and 10-Year Mortality in Elderly European Men and Women: The HALE Project." *Journal of the American Medical Association* 292, no. 12 (2004): 1433–39.

Kwok, C.S. et al. "Habitual Chocolate Consumption and Risk of Cardiovascular Disease Among Healthy Men and Women." *Heart* (online June, 15, 2015): doi: 10.1136/heartjnl-2014-307050.

Lindstedt, I. and Nilsson, P. "Flavanoler, kakao och choklad påverkar hjärt—kärlsystemet" ("Flavanols, Cocoa and Chocolate Affect the Cardiovascular System"). *Läkartidningen* 108 (2011): 324–25.

Liu, S. et al. "Whole-grain Consumption and Risk of Coronary Heart Disease: Results from the Nurses' Health Study." *American Journal of Clinical Nutrition* 70, no. 3 (1999): 412–19.

Nilsson, P.M. "Medelhavskosten skyddar hjärtat" ("Mediterranean Diet Protects the Heart"). *Läkartidningen* 106 (2009): 1959.

Nordic Council of Ministers. *Nutrition Recommendations 2012: Integrating Nutrition and Physical Activity*, 5th edition. Copenhagen: Nord 2014: 002.

Paulun, F. *Blodsockerblues—en bok om glykemiskt index* (*Blood Sugar Blues—A Book About the Glycemic Index*). Stockholm: Fitnessförlaget, 2003.

Rydén, L. et al. "Betala för sjukdom eller investera i hälsa?" ("Pay for Disease or Invest in Health?"). *Läkartidningen* 109 (2012): 1535–39.

Simopoulos, A. "Importance of the Omega-6/Omega-3 Balance in Health and Disease: Evolutionary Aspects of Diet," in *Healthy Agriculture, Healthy Nutrition, Healthy People*, ed. A. Simopoulos. *World Review of Nutrition and Dietetics* 102 (2011): 10–21.

Stender, S. et al. "Ruminant and Industrially Produced Trans Fatty Acids: Health Aspects." *Food & Nutrition Research* 52 (2008): 10.3402/fnr.v52i0.1651.

Stender, S. et al. "Tracing Artificial Trans Fat in Popular Foods in Europe: A Market Basket Investigation." *BMJ Open* 4, no. 5 (2014): e005218.

Swedish National Food Agency. *Swedish Dietary Guidelines*, 2015.

Wolk, A. et al. "A Prospective Study of Association of Mono-unsaturated Fat and Other Types of Fat with Risk of Breast Cancer." *Archives of Internal Medicine* 158, no. 1 (1998): 41–45.

World Cancer Research Fund International. Continuous Update Project, September 2015.

Tip 6. Choose the right drinks

Bhupathiraju, S.N. et al. "Changes in Coffee Intake and Subsequent Risk of Type 2 Diabetes: Three Large Cohorts of US Men and Women." *Diabetologia* 57, no. 7 (2014): 1346–54.

Eskelinen, H.H. et al. "Midlife Coffee and Tea Drinking and the Risk of Late-Life Dementia: A Population-Based CAIDE Study." *Journal of Alzheimer's Disease* 16, no. 1 (2009): 85–91.

Fagrell, B. and Hultcrantz, R. "Alkohol inte enbart av ondo—måttligt intag minskar risk för folksjukdomar" ("Alcohol Not Just Bad—Moderate Consumption Reduces the Risk of Common Diseases"). *Läkartidningen* 109 (2012): 1884–88.

Fredholm, B. "Kaffe minskar risk för Parkinsons sjukdom" ("Coffee Reduces the Risk of Parkinson's Disease"). *Läkartidningen* 101 (2004): 2552–56.

Guercio, B.J. et al. "Coffee Intake, Recurrence, and Mortality in Stage III Colon Cancer: Results From CALGB 89803 (Alliance)." *Journal of Clinical Oncology* 33, no. 31 (2015): 3598–3607.

Hansen, A. "Kaffe minskar risken för stroke" ("Coffee Reduces the Risk of Stroke"). *Läkartidningen* 106 (2009): 919.

Rosendahl, A. et al. "Caffeine and Caffeic Acid Inhibit Growth and Modify Estrogen Receptor and Insulin-Like Growth Factor I Receptor Levels in Human Breast Cancer." *Clinical Cancer Research* 21, no. 8 (2015): 1877–87.

Tip 7. Keep your weight in check

Bengmark, B. "Obesity, the Deadly Quartet and the Contribution of the Neglected Daily Organ Rest—a New Dimension on Un-Health and Its Prevention." *Hepatobiliary Surgery and Nutrition* 4, no. 4 (2015): 278–88.

Swedish Medical Products Agency. "Overweight and Obesity." *Läkemedelsboken (Pharmaceutical book)*. Uppsala: Läkemedelsverket, 2014: 201–208.

Tip 8. Oral health provides general health

Hugoson, A. et al. "Distribution of Peridontal Disease in a Swedish Adult Population 1973, 1983 and 1993." *Journal of Clinical Peridontology* 25 (1998): 542–48.

Hugoson, A. et al. "Oral Health of Individuals Aged 3–80 Years in Jönköping, Sweden During 30 Years (1973–2003). II. Review of Clinical and Radiographic Findings." *Swedish Dental Journal* 29 (2005): 139–55.

Vedin, O. "Prevalence and Prognostic Impact of Peridontal Disease and Conventional Risk Factors in Patients with Stable Coronary Heart Disease." Dissertation, Uppsala University, 2015.

Tip 9. Be an optimist

Chida, Y. and Steptoe, A. "Positive Psychological Well-Being and Mortality: A Quantitative Review of Prospective Observational Studies." *Psychosomatic Medicine* 70, no. 7 (2008): 741–56.

Fexeus, H. *Konsten att få superkrafter (The Art of Gaining Superpowers)*. Stockholm: Forum, 2012, pp. 396–98.

Hernandez, R. et al. "Optimism and Cardiovascular Health: Multi-Ethnic Study of Atherosclerosis (MESA)." *Health Behaviour & Policy Review* 2, no. 1 (2015): 62–73.

Sebö, S. *Bruksanvisning för ett bättre liv (Instructions for a Better Life)*, edition 2.2. Uppsala: Konsultförlaget, 2000.

Tip 10. We need each other

Cole, S. et al. "Myeloid Differential Architecture of Leukocyte Transcriptome Dynamics in Perceived Social Isolation." *Proceedings of the National Academy of Sciences of the United States of America* 112, no. 49 (2015): 15142–47.

Lindmark, A. et al. "Socioeconomic Disparities in Stroke Case Fatality—Observations from Riks-Stroke, the Swedish Stroke Register." *International Journal of Stroke* 9, no. 4 (2014): 429–36.

Valtora, N.K. et al. "Loneliness and Social Isolation as Risk Factors for Coronary Heart Disease and Stroke: Systematic Review and Meta-Analysis of Longitudinal Observational Studies." *Heart* 102, no. 13 (2016): 1009–16.

Wilson, R.S. et al. "Loneliness and Risk of Alzheimer Disease." *Archives of General Psychiatry* 64, no. 2 (2007): 234–40.

THANKS

I HAVE RECEIVED invaluable feedback on this book from:

Johan Appel, Tina Arvidsdotter, Harald Arvidsson, Jenny Bernson, Maria Fredriksson, Sven Kylén, Eva Larsson, Johan Malmquist, Åsa Marklund, Håkan Patrikson, and family members Karin, Martin, and Ola Marklund.

I would also like to thank my daughter Karin Marklund and journalist Nina Olsson for their superb proofreading of the whole text. Thanks also go to my sister, Britt-Inger Henrikson, PhD, for her professional review of the scientific rigor in the book.

Last but not least, I would like to thank Simon Brouwers at Volante and Christine Edhäll at Ahlander Agency for an excellent collaboration and for their fantastic work on this book.

Huge and heartfelt thanks to you all!

BERTIL MARKLUND, VÄNERSBORG, SWEDEN
October 2016